Meditation and its Methods

Swami Vivekananda

INSTITUTE OF THOUGHT & PHILOSOPHY

Published by
GRAPEVINE BOOKS

www.grapevinebooks.com
email: contact@grapevinebooks.com

Ordering Information:
Quantity sales: Special discounts are available on quantity purchases
by corporations, associations, and others.
For details, reach out to the publisher.

First published by Grapevine Books, 2025

Contents

The Importance of Concentration 5

The Development of Concentration 9

Samadhi (Superconsciousness) 12

Non-Attachment 18

Meditation 25

The Power of Meditation 32

The Practice of Meditation 44

Religion As a Practice 50

Mind 57

Controlling The Mind 69

Freedom 73

Freedom is the Goal 80

The End of All Bondage 83

Faith in God 85

Oneness With God 87

The Importance of Concentration

All knowledge that we have, either of the external or internal world, is obtained through only one method — by the concentration of the mind. No knowledge can be had of any science unless we can concentrate our minds upon the subject. The astronomer concentrates his mind through the telescope and so on. If you want to study your own mind, it will be the same process. You will have to concentrate your mind and turn it back upon itself. The difference in this world between mind and mind is simply the fact of concentration. One, more concentrated than the other, gets more knowledge.

Concentration is the essence of all knowledge; nothing can be done without it. Ninety per cent of thought force is wasted by the ordinary human being, and therefore he is constantly committing blunders; the trained man or mind never makes a mistake. Concentration is restraining the mind into smaller and smaller limits.

When the mind is concentrated and turned backward on itself, all within us will be our servants, not our masters. The Greeks applied their concentration to the external world, and the result was perfection in art, literature, etc. The Hindu concentrated on the internal world, upon the unseen realms in the Self, and developed the science of Yoga.

Yoga is controlling the senses, will and mind. The benefit of its study is that we learn to control instead of being controlled.

Mind seems to be layer on layer. Our real goal is to cross all these intervening strata of our being and find God. The end and aim of Yoga is to realise God.

To do this we must go beyond relative knowledge, go beyond the sense-world. The world is awake to the senses, the children of the Lord are asleep on that plane. The world is asleep to the Eternal, the children of the Lord are awake in that realm. These are the sons of God.

There is but one way to control the senses — to see Him who is the Reality in the universe. Then and only then can we really conquer our senses.

The more this power of concentration, the more knowledge is acquired, because this is the one and only method of acquiring knowledge. Even the lowest shoeblack, if he gives more concentration, will black shoes better; the cook with concentration will cook a meal all the better.

In making money, or in worshipping God, or in doing anything, the stronger the power of concentration, the better will that thing be done. This is the one call, the one knock, which opens the gates of nature, and lets out floods of light. This, the power of concentration, is the only key to the treasure-house of knowledge.

*

How are we to know that the mind has become concentrated? Because the idea of time will vanish. The more time passes unnoticed the more concentrated we are.

In common life we see that when we are interested in a book we do not note the time at all; and when we leave the book, we are often surprised to find how many hours have passed. All time will have the tendency to come and stand in the one present.

So the definition is given: When the past and present come and stand in one, the mind is said to be concentrated.

*

We read many books, but that does not bring us knowledge. We may read all the Bibles in the world, but that will not give us religion. Theoretical religion is easy enough to get, any one may get that. What we want is practical religion.

The Christian idea of a practical religion is in doing good works — worldly utility.

What good is utility? Judged from a utilitarian standpoint, religion is a failure. Every hospital is a prayer that more people may come there.

What is meant by charity? Charity is not fundamental. It is really helping on the misery of the world, not eradicating it. One looks for name and fame and covers his efforts to obtain them with the enamel of charity and good works. He is working for himself under the pretext of working for others. Every so-called charity is an encouragement of the very evil it claims to operate against.

Men and women go to balls and dance all night in honour of some hospital or other charitable institution then go home, behave like beasts, and bring devils into the world to fill jails, insane asylums, and hospitals. So it goes on, and it is called good works — building hospital etc.

The ideal of good works is to lessen, or eradicate, the misery of the world. The Yogi says, all misery comes from not being able to control the mind. The Yogi's ideal is freedom from nature. Conquest of nature is his standard of work. The Yogi says that all power is in the soul, and by the controlling of the mind and body one conquers nature by the power of the soul.

*

How has all the knowledge in the world been gained but by the concentration of the powers of the mind? The world is ready to give up its secrets if we only know how to knock, how to give it the necessary blow.

The strength and force of the blow come through concentration. There is no limit to the power of the human mind. The more concentrated it is, the more power is brought to bear on one point; that is the secret.

*

It is impossible to find God outside of ourselves. Our own souls contribute all the divinity that is outside of us. We are the greatest temple. The objectification is only a faint imitation of what we see within ourselves.

Concentration of the powers of the mind is our only instrument to help us see God. If you know one soul (your own), you know all souls, past, present, and to come.

The will concentrates the mind, certain things excite and control this will, such as reason, love, devotion, breathing. The concentrated mind is a lamp that shows us every corner of the soul.

*

The main difference between men and the animals is the difference in their power of concentration. All success in any line of work is the result of this.

Everybody knows something about concentration. We see its results every day. High achievements in art, music, etc., are the results of concentration.

An animal has very little power of concentration. Those who have trained animals find much difficulty in the fact that the animal is constantly forgetting what is told him. He cannot concentrate his mind long upon anything at a time. Herein is the difference between man and the animals — man has the greater power of concentration.

The difference in their power of concentration also constitutes the difference between man and man. Compare the lowest with the highest man. The difference is in the degree of concentration. This is the only difference.

Everybody's mind becomes concentrated at times. We all concentrate upon those things we love, and we love those things upon which we concentrate our minds.

What mother is there that does not love the face of her homeliest child? That face is to her the most beautiful in the world. She loves it because she concentrates her mind on it; and if every one could concentrate his mind on that same face, every one would love it. It would be to all the most beautiful face.

We all concentrate our minds upon those things we love. When we hear beautiful music, our minds become fastened upon it, and we cannot take them away. Those who concentrate their minds upon what you call classical music do not like common music, and vice versa. Music in which the notes follow each other in rapid succession holds the mind readily.

A child loves lively music, because the rapidity of the notes gives the mind no chance to wander. A man who likes common music dislikes classical music, because it is more complicated and requires a greater degree of concentration to follow it.

The great trouble with such concentrations is that we do not control the mind; it controls us. Something outside of ourselves, as it were, draws the mind into it and holds it as long as it chooses. We hear melodious tones or see a beautiful painting, and the mind is held fast! We cannot take it away.

If I speak to you well upon a subject you like, your mind becomes concentrated upon what I am saying. I draw your mind away from yourself and hold it upon the subject in spite of yourself. Thus our attention is held, our minds are concentrated upon various things, in spite of ourselves. We cannot help it.

Now the question is: Can this concentration be developed, and can we become masters of it? The Yogis say, yes. The Yogis say that we can get perfect control of the mind.

On the ethical side there is danger in the development of the power of concentration — the danger of concentrating the mind upon an object and then being unable to detach it at will. This state causes great suffering. Almost all our suffering is caused by our not having the power of detachment.

So along with the development of concentration we must develop the power of detachment. We must learn not only to attach the mind to one thing exclusively, but also to detach it at a moment's notice and place it upon something else. These two should be developed together to make it safe.

This is the systematic development of the mind. To me the very essence of education is concentration of mind, not the collecting of facts. If I had to do my education over again, and had any voice in the matter, I would not study facts at all. I would develop the power of concentration and detachment, and then with a perfect instrument I could collect facts at will. Side by side, in the child, should be developed the power of concentration and detachment.

*

In the lives of all great men, past and present, we find this tremendous power of concentration. Those are men of genius, you say. The science of Yoga tells us that we are all geniuses if we try hard to be. Some will come into this life better fitted and will do it quicker perhaps. We can all do the same. The same power is in everyone. The subject of the present lecture is how to concentrate the mind in order to study the mind itself. Yogis have laid down certain rules and this night I am going to give you a sketch of some of these rules.

The Development of Concentration

Concentration, of course, comes from various sources. Through the senses you can get concentration. Some get it when they hear beautiful music, others when they see beautiful scenery. Some get concentrated by lying upon beds of spikes, sharp iron spikes, others by sitting upon sharp pebbles.

These are extraordinary cases [using] most unscientific procedure. Scientific procedure is gradually training the mind.

One gets concentrated by holding his arm up. Torture gives him the concentration he wants. But all these are extraordinary.

Universal methods have been organised according to different philosophers. Some say the state we want to attain is super-consciousness of the mind — going beyond the limitations the body has made for us.

The value of ethics to the Yogi lies in that it makes the mind pure. The purer the mind, the easier it is to control it. The mind takes every thought that rises and works it out. The grosser the mind, the more difficult [it is] to control [it].

The immoral man will never be able to concentrate his mind to study psychology. He may get a little control as he begins, get a little power of hearing. and even those powers will go from him. The difficulty is that if you study closely, you see how [the] extraordinary power arrived at was not attained by regular scientific training.

The men who, by the power of magic, control serpents will be killed by serpents. The man who attains any extraordinary powers will in the long run succumb to those powers. There are millions [who] receive power through all sorts of ways in India. The vast majority of them die raving lunatics. Quite a number commit suicide, the mind [being] unbalanced.

The study must be put on the safe side: scientific, slow, peaceful. The first requisite is to be moral. Such a man wants the gods to come down, and they will come down and manifest themselves to him. That is our psychology and philosophy in essence, [to be] perfectly moral.

Just think what that means! No injury, perfect purity, perfect austerity! These are absolutely necessary. Just think, if a man can attain all these in perfection! What more do you want? If he is free from all enmity towards any being, all animals will give up their enmity [in his presence].

*

The law of laws is concentration. First, concentrate all the nerve energies and all power lodged in the cells of the body into one force and direct it at will. Then bring the mind, which is thinner matter, into one centre.

The mind has layer after layer. When the nerve force concentrated is made to pass through the spinal column, one layer of the mind is open. When it is concentrated in one bone [plexus, or "lotus"], another part of the world is open.

So from world to world it goes until it touches the pineal gland in the centre of the brain. This is the seat of conservation of potential energy, the source of both activity and passivity.

*

No one method can suit all. Different methods are not steps necessary to be taken one after another. Ceremonials are the lowest form; next God external, and after that God internal.

In some cases gradation may be needed, but in many only one way is required. It would be the height of folly to say to everyone, "You must pass through Karma and Bhakti before you can reach Jnana."

Stick to your reason until you reach something higher; and you will know it to be higher, because it will not jar with reason. The stage beyond consciousness is inspiration (Samâdhi); but never mistake hysterical trances for the real thing.

It is a terrible thing to claim this inspiration falsely, to mistake instinct for inspiration. There is no external test for inspiration, we know it ourselves; our guardian against mistake is negative — the voice of reason. All religion is going beyond reason, but reason is the only guide to get there.

Instinct is like ice, reason is the water, and inspiration is the subtlest form or vapour; one follows the other. Everywhere is this eternal sequence — unconsciousness, consciousness, intelligence — matter, body, mind — and to us it seems as if the chain began with the particular link we first lay hold of.

Arguments on both sides are of equal weight, and both are true. We must reach beyond both, to where there is neither the one nor the other. These successions are all Maya.

*

It is easy to concentrate the mind on external things, the mind naturally goes outwards; but not so in the case of religion, or psychology, or metaphysics, where the subject and the object, are one. The object is internal, the mind itself is the object, and it is necessary to study the mind itself — mind studying mind.

We know that there is the power of the mind called reflection. I am talking to you. At the same time I am standing aside, as it were, a second person, and knowing and hearing what I am talking. You work and think at the same time, while a portion of your mind stands by and sees what you are thinking.

The powers of the mind should be concentrated and turned back upon itself, and as the darkest places reveal their secrets before the penetrating rays of the sun, so will this concentrated mind penetrate its own innermost secrets. Thus will we come to the basis of belief, the real genuine religion. We will perceive for ourselves whether we have souls, whether life is of five minutes or of eternity, whether there is a God in the universe or more. It will all be revealed to us.

This is what Raja-Yoga proposes to teach. The goal of all its teaching is how to concentrate the minds, then, how to discover the innermost recesses of our own minds, then, how to generalise their contents and form our own conclusions from them.

It, therefore, never asks the question what our religion is, whether we are Deists or Atheists, whether Christians, Jews, or Buddhists. We are human beings; that is sufficient. Every human being has the right and the power to seek for religion. Every human being has the right to ask the reason, why, and to have his question answered by himself, if he only takes the trouble.

So far, then, we see that in the study of this Raja-Yoga no faith or belief is necessary. Believe nothing until you find it out for yourself; that is what it teaches us.

*

Do you mean to say that the facts of our awakened state require any dreams or imaginings to prove them? Certainly not. This study of Raja-Yoga takes a long time and constant practice. A part of this practice is physical, but in the main it is mental.

As we proceed we shall find how intimately the mind is connected with the body. If we believe that the mind is simply a finer part of the body, and that mind acts upon the body, then it stands to reason that the body must react upon the mind.

If the body is sick, the mind becomes sick also. If the body is healthy, the mind remains healthy and strong. When one is angry, the mind becomes disturbed. Similarly when the mind is disturbed, the body also becomes disturbed.

With the majority of mankind the mind is greatly under the control of the body, their mind being very little developed. The vast mass of humanity is very little removed from the animals. Not only so, but in many instances, the power of control in them is little higher than that of the lower animals.

We have very little command of our minds. Therefore to bring that command about, to get that control over body and mind, we must take certain physical helps. When the body is sufficiently controlled, we can attempt the manipulation of the mind.

By manipulating the mind, we shall be able to bring it under our control, make it work as we like, and compel it to concentrate its powers as we desire.

Samadhi (Superconsciousness)

All our knowledge which is called rational is referred to consciousness. My consciousness of this table, and of your presence, makes me know that the table and you are here. At the same time, there is a very great part of my existence of which I am not conscious. All the different organs inside the body, the different parts of the brain — nobody is conscious of these.

When I eat food, I do it consciously; when I assimilate it, I do it unconsciously. When the food is manufactured into blood, it is done unconsciously. When out of the blood all the different parts of my body are strengthened, it is done unconsciously.

And yet it is I who am doing all this; there cannot be twenty people in this one body. How do I know that I do it, and nobody else? It may be urged that my business is only in eating and assimilating the food, and that strengthening the body by the food is done for me by somebody else.

That cannot be, because it can be demonstrated that almost every action of which we are now unconscious can be brought up to the plane of consciousness. The heart is beating apparently without our control. None of us here can control the heart; it goes on its own way.

But by practice men can bring even the heart under control, until it will just beat at will, slowly, or quickly, or almost stop. Nearly every part of the body can be brought under control.

*

What does this show? That the functions which are beneath consciousness are also performed by us, only we are doing it unconsciously.

We have, then, two planes in which the human mind works. First is the conscious plane, in which all work is always accompanied with the feeling of egoism. Next comes the unconscious plane, where all work is unaccompanied by the feeling of egoism.

That part of mind-work which is unaccompanied with the feeling of egoism is unconscious work, and that part which is accompanied with the feeling of egoism is conscious work. In the lower animals this unconscious work is called instinct. In higher animals, and in the highest of all animals, man, what is called conscious work prevails.

*

But it does not end here. There is a still higher plane upon which the mind can work. It can go beyond consciousness. Just as unconscious work is beneath consciousness, so there is another work which is above consciousness, and which also is not accompanied with the feeling of egoism.

The feeling of egoism is only on the middle plane. When the mind is above or below that line, there is no feeling of "I", and yet the mind works. When the mind goes beyond this line of self-consciousness, it is called Samâdhi or superconsciousness.

How, for instance, do we know that a man in Samadhi has not gone below consciousness, has not degenerated instead of going higher? In both cases the works are unaccompanied with egoism.

The answer is, by the effects, by the results of the work, we know that which is below, and that which is above. When a man goes into deep sleep, he enters a plane beneath consciousness. He works the body all the time, he breathes, he moves the body, perhaps, in his sleep, without any accompanying feeling of ego; he is unconscious, and when he returns from his sleep, he is the same man who went into it.

The sum total of the knowledge which he had before he went into the sleep remains the same; it does not increase at all. No enlightenment comes. But when a man goes into Samadhi, if he goes into it a fool, he comes out a sage.

What makes the difference? From one state a man comes out the very same man that he went in, and from another state the man comes out enlightened, a sage, a prophet, a saint, his whole character changed, his life changed, illumined. These are the two effects. Now the effects being different, the causes must be different. As this illumination with which a man comes back from Samadhi is much higher than can be got from unconsciousness, or much higher than can be got by reasoning in a conscious state, it must, therefore, be superconsciousness, and Samadhi is called the superconscious state.

*

This, in short, is the idea of Samadhi. What is its application?

The application is here. The field of reason, or of the conscious workings of the mind, is narrow and limited. There is a little circle within which human reason must move. It cannot go beyond. Every attempt to go beyond is impossible, yet it is beyond this circle of reason that there lies all that humanity holds most dear.

All these questions, whether there is an immortal soul, whether there is a God, whether there is any supreme intelligence guiding this universe or not, are beyond the field of reason. Reason can never answer these questions. What does reason say? It says, "I am agnostic; I do not know either yea or nay."

Yet these questions are so important to us. Without a proper answer to them, human life will be purposeless. All our ethical theories, all our moral attitudes, all that is good and great in human nature, have been moulded upon answers that have come from beyond the circle.

It is very important, therefore, that we should have answers to these questions. If life is only a short play, if the universe is only a "fortuitous combination of atoms," then why should I do good to another? Why should there be mercy, justice, or fellow-feeling? The best thing for this world would be to make hay while the sun shines, each man for himself.

If there is no hope, why should I love my brother, and not cut his throat? If there is nothing beyond, if there is no freedom, but only rigorous dead laws, I should only try to make myself happy here.

You will find people saying nowadays that they have utilitarian grounds as the basis of morality. What is this basis? Procuring the greatest amount of happiness to the greatest number. Why should I do this? Why should I not produce the greatest unhappiness to the greatest number, if that serves my purpose? How will utilitarians answer this question? How do you know what is right, or what is wrong?

I am impelled by my desire for happiness, and I fulfil it, and it is in my nature; I know nothing beyond. I have these desires, and must fulfil them; why should you complain? Whence come all these truths about human life, about morality, about the immortal soul, about God, about love and sympathy, about being good, and, above all, about being unselfish?

All ethics, all human action and all human thought, hang upon this one idea of unselfishness. The whole idea of human life can be put into that one word, unselfishness.

Why should we be unselfish? Where is the necessity, the force, the power, of my being unselfish?

You call yourself a rational man, a utilitarian; but if you do not show me a reason for utility, I say you are irrational. Show me the reason why I should not be selfish. To ask one to be unselfish may be good as poetry, but poetry is not reason. Show me a reason.

Why shall I be unselfish, and why be good? Because Mr. and Mrs. So-and-so say so does not weigh with me. Where is the utility of my being unselfish? My utility is to be selfish if utility means the greatest amount of happiness. What is the answer? The utilitarian can never give it.

*

The answer is that this world is only one drop in an infinite ocean, one link in an infinite chain. Where did those that preached unselfishness, and taught it to the human race, get this idea? We know it is not instinctive; the animals, which have instinct, do not know it. Neither is it reason; reason does not know anything about these ideas. Whence then did they come?

We find, in studying history, one fact held in common by all the great teachers of religion the world ever had. They all claim to have got their truths from beyond, only many of them did not know where they got them from.

For instance, one would say that an angel came down in the form of a human being, with wings, and said to him, "Hear, O man, this is the message." Another says that a Deva, a bright being, appeared to him.

A third says he dreamed that his ancestor came and told him certain things. He did not know anything beyond that. But this is common that all claim that this knowledge has come to them from beyond, not through their reasoning power.

What does the science of Yoga teach? It teaches that they were right in claiming that all this knowledge came to them from beyond reasoning, but that it came from within themselves.

The Yogi teaches that the mind itself has a higher state of existence, beyond reason, a superconscious state, and when the mind gets to that higher state, then this knowledge, beyond reasoning, comes to man. Metaphysical and transcendental knowledge comes to that man.

This state of going beyond reason, transcending ordinary human nature, may sometimes come by chance to a man who does not understand its science; he, as it were, stumbles upon it. When he stumbles upon it, he generally interprets it as coming from outside. So this explains why an inspiration, or transcendental knowledge, may be the same in different countries, but in one country it will seem to come through an angel, and in another through a Deva, and in a third through God.

What does it mean? It means that the mind brought the knowledge by its own nature, and that the finding of the knowledge was interpreted according to the belief and education of the person through whom it came. The real fact is that these various men, as it were, stumbled upon this superconscious state.

The Yogi says there is a great danger in stumbling upon this state. In a good many cases there is the danger of the brain being deranged, and, as a rule, you will find that all those men, however great they were, who had stumbled upon this superconscious state without understanding it, groped in the dark, and generally had, along with their knowledge, some quaint superstition. They opened themselves to hallucinations.

Mohammed claimed that the Angel Gabriel came to him in a cave one day and took him on the heavenly horse, Harak, and he visited the heavens. But with all that, Mohammed spoke some wonderful truths. If you read the Koran, you find the most wonderful truths mixed with superstitions.

How will you explain it? That man was inspired, no doubt, but that inspiration was, as it were, stumbled upon. He was not a trained Yogi, and did not know the reason of what he was doing.

Think of the good Mohammed did to the world, and think of the great evil that has been done through his fanaticism! Think of the millions massacred through his teachings, mothers bereft of their children, children made orphans, whole countries destroyed, millions upon millions of people killed!

So we see this danger by studying the lives of great teachers like Mohammed and others. Yet we find, at the same time, that they were all inspired. Whenever a prophet got into the superconscious state by heightening his emotional nature, he brought away from it not only some truths, but some fanaticism also, some superstition which injured the world as much as the greatness of the teaching helped.

To get any reason out of the mass of incongruity we call human life, we have to transcend our reason, but we must do it scientifically, slowly, by regular practice, and we must cast off all superstition. We must take up the study of the superconscious state just as any other science. On reason we must have to lay our foundation, we must follow reason as far as it leads, and when reason fails, reason itself will show us the way to the highest plane.

When you hear a man say, "I am inspired," and then talk irrationally, reject it. Why? Because these three states — instinct, reason, and super-consciousness, or the unconscious, conscious, and superconscious states — belong to one and the same mind. There are not three minds in one man, but one state of it develops into the others. Instinct develops into reason, and reason into the transcendental consciousness; therefore, not one of the states contradicts the others.

Real inspiration never contradicts reason, but fulfils it. Just as you find the great prophets saying, "I come not to destroy but to fulfil," so inspiration always comes to fulfil reason, and is in harmony with it.

*

All the different steps in Yoga are intended to bring us scientifically to the superconscious state, or Samadhi. Furthermore, this is a most vital point to understand, that inspiration is as much in every man's nature as it was in that of the ancient prophets.

These prophets were not unique; they were men as you or I. They were great Yogis. They had gained this super-consciousness, and you and I can get the same. They were not peculiar people. The very fact that one man ever reached that state, proves that it is possible for every man to do so. Not only is it possible, but every man must, eventually, get to that state, and that is religion.

Experience is the only teacher we have. We may talk and reason all our lives, but we shall not understand a word of truth, until we experience it ourselves.

You cannot hope to make a man a surgeon by simply giving him a few books. You cannot satisfy my curiosity to see a country by showing me a map; I must have actual experience. Maps can only create curiosity in us to get more perfect knowledge. Beyond that, they have no value whatever.

Clinging to books only degenerates the human mind. Was there ever a more horrible blasphemy than the statement that all the knowledge of God is confined to this or that book? How dare men call God infinite, and yet try to compress Him within the covers of a little book!

Millions of people have been killed because they did not believe what the books said, because they would not see all the knowledge of God within the covers of a book. Of course, this killing and murdering has gone by, but the world is still tremendously bound up in a belief in books.

*

When the mind has been trained to remain fixed on a certain internal or external location, there comes to it the power of flowing in an unbroken current, as it were, towards that point. This state is called Dhyana.

When one has so intensified the power of Dhyana as to be able to reject the external part of perception and remain meditating only on the internal part, the meaning, that state is called Samadhi.

That is, if the mind can first concentrate upon an object, and then is able to continue in that concentration for a length of time, and then, by continued concentration, to dwell only on the internal part of the perception of which the object was the effect, everything comes under the control of such a mind.

This meditative state is the highest state of existence. So long as there is desire, no real happiness can come. It is only the contemplative, witness-like study of objects that brings to us real enjoyment and happiness. The animal has its happiness in the senses, the man in his intellect, and the god in spiritual contemplation.

It is only to the soul that has attained to this contemplative state that the world really becomes beautiful. To him who desires nothing, and does not mix himself up with them, the manifold changes of nature are one panorama of beauty and sublimity.

Non-Attachment

Does renunciation demand that we all become ascetics? Who then is to help others? Renunciation is not asceticism. Are all beggars Christ? Poverty is not a synonym for holiness; often the reverse.

Renunciation is of the mind. How does it come? In a desert, when I was thirsty, I saw a lake. It was in the midst of a beautiful landscape. There were trees surrounding it, and their reflections could be seen in the water, upside down. But the whole thing proved to be a mirage.

Then I knew that every day for a month I had seen this; and only that day, being thirsty, I had learnt it to be unreal. Every day for a month I should see it again. But I should never take it to be real.

So, when we reach God, the idea of the universe, the body and so on, will vanish. It will return afterwards. But next time we shall know it to be unreal.

The history of the world is the history of persons like Buddha and Jesus. The passionless and unattached do most for the world.

Picture Jesus in the slums. He sees beyond the misery, "You, my brethren, are all divine." His work is calm. He removes causes. You will be able to work for the good of the world when you know for a fact that this work is all illusion.

The more unconscious this work, the better, because it is then the more superconscious. Our search is not for good or evil; but happiness and good are nearer to truth than their opposites.

A man ran a thorn into his finger, and with another thorn took it out. The first thorn is Evil. The second thorn is Good. The Self is that Peace which passeth beyond both evil and good.

The universe is melting down: man draws nearer to God. For one moment he is real — God. He is re-differentiated — a prophet. Before him, now, the world trembles. A fool sleeps and wakes a fool-a man unconscious; and superconscious, he returns with infinite power, purity, and love — the God-Man. This is the use of the superconscious state.

*

Attachment is the source of all our pleasures now. We are attached to our friends, to our relatives; we are attached to our intellectual and spiritual works; we are attached to external objects, so that we get pleasure from them.

What, again, brings misery but this very attachment? We have to detach ourselves to earn joy. If only we had power to detach ourselves at will, there would not be any misery. That man alone will be able to get the best of nature, who, having the power of attaching himself to a thing with all his energy, has also the power to detach himself when he should do so.

The difficulty is that there must be as much power of attachment as that of detachment. There are men who are never attracted by anything. They can never love, they are hard-hearted and apathetic; they escape most of the miseries of life.

But the wall never feels misery, the wall never loves, is never hurt; but it is the wall, after all. Surely it is better to be attached and caught, than to be a wall. Therefore the man who never loves, who is hard and stony, escaping most of the miseries of life, escapes also its joys.

We do not want that. That is weakness, that is death. That soul has not been awakened that never feels weakness, never feels misery. That is a callous state. We do not want that.

At the same time, we not only want this mighty power of love, this mighty power of attachment, the power of throwing our whole soul upon a single object, losing ourselves and letting ourselves be annihilated, as it were, for other souls — which is the power of the gods — but we want to be higher even than the gods.

The perfect man can put his whole soul upon that one point of love, yet he is unattached. How comes this? There is another secret to learn.

The beggar is never happy. The beggar only gets a dole with pity and scorn behind it, at least with the thought behind that the beggar is a low object. He never really enjoys what he gets.

We are all beggars. Whatever we do, we want a return. We are all traders. We are traders in life, we are traders in virtue, we are traders in religion. And alas! we are also traders in love.

If you come to trade, if it is a question of give-and-take, if it is a question of buy-and-sell, abide by the laws of buying and selling. There is a bad time and there is a good time; there is a rise and a fall in prices: always you expect the blow to come.

It is like looking at the mirrors Your face is reflected: you make a grimace — there is one in the mirror; if you laugh, the mirror laughs. This is buying and selling, giving and taking.

We get caught. How? Not by what we give, but by what we expect. We get misery in return for our love; not from the fact that we love, but from the fact that we want love in return.

There is no misery where there is no want. Desire, want, is the father of all misery. Desires are bound by the laws of success and failure. Desires must bring misery.

*

The great secret of true success, of true happiness, then, is this: the man who asks for no return, the perfectly unselfish man, is the most successful.

It seems to be a paradox. Do we not know that every man who is unselfish in life gets cheated, gets hurt? Apparently, yes. "Christ was unselfish, and yet he was crucified."

True, but we know that his unselfishness is the reason, the cause of a great victory —

the crowning of millions upon millions of lives with the blessings of true success.

Ask nothing; want nothing in return. Give what you have to give; it will come back to you — but do not think of that now, it will come back multiplied a thousandfold — but the attention must not be on that. Yet have the power to give: give, and there it ends. Learn that the whole of life is giving, that nature will force you to give.

So, give willingly. Sooner or later you will have to give up. You come into life to accumulate. With clenched hands, you want to take. But nature puts a hand on your throat and makes your hands open.

Whether you will it or not, you have to give. The moment you say, "I will not", the blow comes; you are hurt. None is there but will be compelled, in the long run, to give up everything. And the more one struggles against this law, the more miserable one feels.

It is because we dare not give, because we are not resigned enough to accede to this grand demand of nature, that we are miserable. The forest is gone, but we get heat in return. The sun is taking up water from the ocean, to return it in showers. You are a machine for taking and giving: you take, in order to give.

Ask, therefore, nothing in return; but the more you give, the more will come to you. The quicker you can empty the air out of this room, the quicker it will be filled up by the external air; and if you close all the doors and every aperture, that which is within will remain, but that which is outside will never come in, and that which is within will stagnate, degenerate, and become poisoned.

A river is continually emptying itself into the ocean and is continually filling up again. Bar not the exit into the ocean. The moment you do that, death seizes you.

*

Be, therefore, not a beggar; be unattached.

This is the most terrible task of life! You do not calculate the dangers on the path. Even by intellectually recognising the difficulties, we really do not know them until we feel them. From a distance we may get a general view of a park: well, what of that? We feel and really know it when we are in it. Even if our every attempt is a failure, and we bleed and are torn asunder, yet, through all this, we have to preserve our heart — we must assert our Godhead in the midst of all these difficulties.

Nature wants us to react, to return blow for blow, cheating for cheating, lie for lie, to hit back with all our might. Then it requires a superdivine power not to hit back, to keep control, to be unattached.

Every day we renew our determination to be unattached. We cast our eyes back and look at the past objects of our love and attachment, and feel how every one of them made us miserable. We went down into the depths of despondency because of our "love"! We found ourselves mere slaves in the hands of others, we were dragged down and down!

And we make a fresh determination: "Henceforth, I will be master of myself;

henceforth, I will have control over myself." But the time comes, and the same story once more! Again the soul is caught and cannot get out. The bird is in a net, struggling and fluttering. This is our life.

I know the difficulties. Tremendous they are, and ninety per cent of us become discouraged and lose heart, and in our turn, often become pessimists and cease to believe in sincerity, love, and all that is grand and noble.

So, we find men who in the freshness of their lives have been forgiving, kind, simple, and guileless, become in old age lying masks of men. Their minds are a mass of intricacy.

There may be a good deal of external policy, possibly. They are not hot-headed, they do not speak, but it would be better for them to do so; their hearts are dead and, therefore, they do not speak. They do not curse, not become angry; but it would be better for them to be able to be angry, a thousand times better, to be able to curse. They cannot. There is death in the heart, for cold hands have seized upon it, and it can no more act, even to utter a curse, even to use a harsh word.

All this we have to avoid: therefore I say, we require superdivine power. Superhuman power is not strong enough. Superdivine strength is the only way, the one way out. By it alone we can pass through all these intricacies, through these showers of miseries, unscathed. We may be cut to pieces, torn asunder, yet our hearts must grow nobler and nobler all the time.

It is very difficult, but we can overcome the difficulty by constant practice. We must learn that nothing can happen to us, unless we make ourselves susceptible to it.

*

I have just said, no disease can come to me until the body is ready; it does not depend alone on the germs, but upon a certain predisposition which is already in the body. We get only that for which we are fitted.

Let us give up our pride and understand this, that never is misery undeserved. There never has been a blow undeserved: there never has been an evil for which I did not pave the way with my own hands. We ought to know that.

Analyse yourselves and you will find that every blow you have received, came to you because you prepared yourselves for it. You did half, and the external world did the other half: that is how the blow came. That will sober us down.

At the same time, from this very analysis will come a note of hope, and the note of hope is: "I have no control of the external world, but that which is in me and nearer unto me, my own world, is in my control. If the two together are required to make a failure, if the two together are necessary to give me a blow, I will not contribute the one which is in my keeping; and how then can the blow come? If I get real control of myself, the blow will never come."

*

By non-attachment and practice, meditation is perfected.

*

"I cannot tell anything about Thee except that Thou art my love. Thou art beautiful, Oh, Thou art beautiful! Thou art beauty itself." What is after all really required of us in this Yoga is that our thirst after the beautiful should be directed to God.

What is the beauty in the human face, in the sky, in the stars, and in the moon? It is only the partial apprehension of the real all-embracing Divine Beauty. "He shining, everything shines. It is through His light that all things shine."

Take this high position of Bhakti which makes you forget at once all your little personalities. Take yourself away from all the world's little selfish clingings. Do not look upon humanity as the centre of all your human and higher interests. Stand as a witness, as a student, and observe the phenomena of nature. Have the feeling of personal non-attachment with regard to man, and see how this mighty feeling of love is working itself out in the world.

Sometimes a little friction is produced, but that is only in the course of the struggle to attain the higher real love. Sometimes there is a little fight or a little fall; but it is all only by the way.

Stand aside, and freely let these frictions come. You feel the frictions only when you are in the current of the world, but when you are outside of it simply as a witness and as a student, you will be able to see that there are millions and millions of channels in which God is manifesting Himself as Love.

*

The Bhakti-Yogi knows the meaning of life's struggles; he understands it. He has passed through a long series of these struggles and knows what they mean and earnestly desires to be free from the friction thereof; he wants to avoid the clash and go direct to the centre of all attraction, the great Hari.

This is the renunciation of the Bhakta. This mighty attraction in the direction of God makes all other attractions vanish for him. This mighty infinite love of God which enters his heart leaves no place for any other love to live there.

How can it be otherwise? Bhakti fills his heart with the divine waters of the ocean of love, which is God Himself; there is no place there for little loves. That is to say, the Bhakta's renunciation is that Vairâgya or non-attachment for all things that are not God which results from Anurâga or great attachment to God.

*

Whenever we say a thing is "mine", misery will immediately come. Do not even say "my child" in your mind. Possess the child, but do not say "mine". If you do, then will come the misery.

Do not say "my house," do not say "my body". The whole difficulty is there. The body is neither yours, nor mine, nor anybody's. These bodies are coming and going by the laws of nature, but we are free, standing as witness.

This body is no more free than a picture or a wall. Why should we be attached so much to a body? If somebody paints a picture, he does it and passes on. Do not project that tentacle of selfishness, "I must possess it". As soon as that is projected, misery will begin.

So Karma-Yoga says, first destroy the tendency to project this tentacle of selfishness, and when you have the power of checking it, hold it in and do not allow the mind to get into the ways of selfishness. Then you may go out into the world and work as much as you can. Mix everywhere, go where you please; you will never be contaminated with evil. There is the lotus leaf in the water; the water cannot touch and adhere to it; so will you be in the world. This is called "Vairâgya", dispassion or non-attachment.

I believe I have told you that without non-attachment there cannot be any kind of Yoga. Non-attachment is the basis of all the Yogas. The man who gives up living in houses, wearing fine clothes, and eating good food, and goes into the desert, may be a most attached person. His only possession, his own body, may become everything to him; and as he lives he will be simply struggling for the sake of his body.

Non-attachment does not mean anything that we may do in relation to our external body, it is all in the mind. The binding link of "I and mine" is in the mind. If we have not this link with the body and with the things of the senses, we are non-attached, wherever and whatever we may be. A man may be on a throne and perfectly non-attached; another man may be in rags and still very much attached.

First, we have to attain this state of non-attachment and then to work incessantly. Karma-Yoga gives us the method that will help us in giving up all attachment, though it is indeed very hard.

*

The body is our enemy, and yet is our friend. Which of you can bear the sight of misery? And which of you cannot do so when you see it only as a painting? Because it is unreal, we do not identify ourselves with it, eve know it is only a painting; it cannot bless us, it cannot hurt us.

The most terrible misery painted upon a price of canvas, we may even enjoy; we praise the technique of the artist, we wonder at his marvellous genius, even though the scene he paints is most horrible. That is the secret; that non-attachment. Be the Witness.

*

Since I was a child I have heard about Krishna's life. I take it for granted there must have been a man called Krishna, and his Gita shows he has [left] a wonderful book.

I told you, you can understand the character of a man by analysing the fables about him. The fables have the nature [of decorations]. You must find they are all polished and manipulated to fit into the character.

For instance, take Buddha. The central idea [is] sacrifice. There are thousands of folklore, but in every case the sacrifice must have been kept up.

There are thousands of stories about Lincoln, about some characteristic of that great man. You take all the fables and find the general idea and [know] that that was the central character of the man.

You find in Krishna that non-attachment is the central idea. He does not need anything. He does not want anything. He works for work's sake. "Work for work's sake. Worship for worship's sake. Do good because it is good to do good. Ask no more."

That must have been the character of the man. Otherwise these fables could not be brought down to the one idea of non-attachment.

*

The purer the body and mind, the quicker the desired result will be obtained. You must be perfectly pure. Do not think of evil things, such thoughts will surely drag you down.

If you are perfectly pure and practice faithfully, your mind can finally be made a searchlight of infinite power. There is no limit to its scope.

But there must be constant practice and non-attachment to the world. When a man reaches the superconscious state, all feeling of body melts away. Then alone does he become free and immortal.

Meditation

We are at the beck and call of nature. If there is sound outside, I have to hear it. If something is going on, I have to see it. Like monkeys. We are two thousand monkeys concentrated, each one of us.

Monkeys are very curious. So we cannot help ourselves, and call this "enjoying". Wonderful this language! We are enjoying the world! We cannot help enjoying it. Nature wants us to do it. A beautiful sound: I am hearing it. As if I could choose to hear it or not!

Nature says, "Go down to the depths of misery." I become miserable in a moment. We talk about pleasures [of the senses] and possessions.

One man thinks me very learned. Another thinks, "He is a fool." This degradation, this slavery, without knowing anything! In the dark room we are knocking our heads against each other.

What is meditation? Meditation is the power which enables us to resist all this.

Nature may call us, "Look there is a beautiful thing!" I do not look. Now she says, "There is a beautiful smell; smell it! " I say to my nose, "Do not smell it", and the nose doesn't. "Eyes, do not see!"

Nature does such an awful thing - kills one of my children, and says, "Now, rascal, sit down and weep! Go to the depths!" I say, "I don't have to." I jump up. I must be free.

Try it sometimes. [In meditation], for a moment, you can change this nature. Now, if you had that power in yourself, would not that be heaven, freedom? That is the power of meditation.

*

Always think that this body is only an inert instrument. And the self-contained Purusha within is your real nature. The adjunct of mind is His first and subtle covering, then, there is this body which is His gross, outer covering. The indivisible changeless, self-effulgent Purusha is lying hidden under these delusive veils, therefore your real nature is unknown to you.

The direction of the mind which always runs after the senses has to be turned within. The mind has to be killed. The body is but gross — it dies and dissolves into the five elements.

But the bundle of mental impressions, which is the mind, does not die soon. It remains for some time in seed-form and then sprouts and grows in the form of a tree — it takes on another physical body and goes the round of birth and death, until Self-knowledge arises.

Therefore I say, by meditation and concentration and by the power of philosophical discrimination plunge this mind in the Ocean of Existence-Knowledge-Bliss Absolute. When the mind dies, all limiting adjuncts vanish and you are established in Brahman.

*

First, meditation should be of a negative nature. Think away everything. Analyse everything that comes in the mind by the sheer action of the will.

Next, assert what we really are — existence, knowledge and bliss — being, knowing, and loving.

Meditation is the means of unification of the subject and object. Meditate:

Above, it is full of me; below, it is full of me; in the middle, it is full of me. I am in all beings, and all beings are in me. Om Tat Sat, I am It. I am existence above mind. I am the one Spirit of the universe. I am neither pleasure nor pain.

The body drinks, eats, and so on. I am not the body. I am not mind. I am He.

I am the witness. I look on. When health comes I am the witness When disease comes I am the witness.

I am Existence, Knowledge, Bliss.

I am the essence and nectar of knowledge. Through eternity I change not. I am calm, resplendent, and unchanging.

*

Be like the pearl oyster. There is a pretty Indian fable to the effect that if it rains when the star Svâti is in the ascendant, and a drop of rain falls into an oyster, that drop becomes a pearl.

The oysters know this, so they come to the surface when that star shines, and wait to catch the precious raindrop. When a drop falls into them, quickly the oysters close their shells and dive down to the bottom of the sea, there to patiently develop the drop into the pearl.

We should be like that. First hear, then understand, and then, leaving all distractions, shut your minds to outside influences, and devote yourselves to developing the truth within you.

There is the danger of frittering away your energies by taking up an idea only for its novelty, and then giving it up for another that is newer. Take one thing up and do it, and see the end of it, and before you have seen the end, do not give it up.

He who can become mad with an idea, he alone sees light. Those that only take a nibble here and a nibble there will never attain anything. They may titillate their nerves for a moment, but there it will end. They will be slaves in the hands of nature, and will never get beyond the senses.

*

Those who really want to be Yogis must give up, once for all, this nibbling at things. Take up one idea. Make that one idea your life — think of it, dream of it, live on that idea. Let the brain, muscles, nerves, every part of your body, be full of that idea, and just leave every other idea alone.

This is the way to success, and this is the way great spiritual giants are produced. Others are mere talking machines. If we really want to be blessed, and make others blessed, we must go deeper.

The first step is not to disturb the mind, not to associate with persons whose ideas are disturbing. All of you know that certain persons, certain places, certain foods, repel you. Avoid them; and those who want to go to the highest, must avoid all company, good or bad.

Practise hard; whether you live or die does not matter. You have to plunge in and work, without thinking of the result. If you are brave enough, in six months you will be a perfect Yogi.

But those who take up just a bit of it and a little of everything else make no progress. It is of no use simply to take a course of lessons. To those who are full of Tamas, ignorant and dull — those whose minds never get fixed on any idea, who only crave for something to amuse them — religion and philosophy are simply objects of entertainment. These are the unpersevering. They hear a talk, think it very nice, and then go home and forget all about it.

To succeed, you must have tremendous perseverance, tremendous will. "I will drink the ocean," says the persevering soul, "at my will mountains will crumble up." Have that sort of energy, that sort of will, work hard, and you will reach the goal.

*

There is one soul which is the greatest of all. This is Ishvara, Lord of Yoga [God as Creator, with attributes]. He is the individual. He is omnipotent. He resides in every heart.

There is no body. He does not need a body. All you get by the practice of meditation etc., you can get by meditation upon Ishvara, Lord of Yogis.

The same can be attained by meditating upon a great soul; or upon the harmony of life. These are called objective meditations.

So, you begin to meditate upon certain external things, objective things, either outside or inside. If you take a long sentence, that is no meditation at all. That is simply trying to get the mind collected by repetition.

Meditation means the mind is turned back upon itself. The mind stops all the [thought-waves] and the world stops. Your consciousness expands. Every time you meditate you will keep your growth.

Work a little harder, more and more, and meditation comes. You do not feel the body or anything else. When you come out of it after the hour, you have had the most beautiful rest you ever had in your life. That is the only way you ever give rest to your system. Not even the deepest sleep will give you such rest as that.

The mind goes on jumping even in deepest sleep. Just those few minutes [in meditation] your brain has almost stopped. Just a little vitality is kept up.

You may be cut to pieces and not feel it at all. You feel such pleasure in it. You become so light. This perfect rest we will get in meditation.

*

Meditation is a sort of prayer and prayer is meditation. The highest meditation is to think of nothing. If you can remain one moment without thought, great power will come. The whole secret of knowledge is concentration.

Soul best develops itself by loving God with all the heart. Soul is the thinking principle in man, of which mind is a function. Soul is only the conduit from Spirit to mind.

*

These ideas have to be understood in Dhyana, or meditation. We hear a sound. First, there is the external vibration; second, the nerve motion that carries it to the mind; third, the reaction from the mind, along with which flashes the knowledge of the object which was the external cause of these different changes from the ethereal vibrations to the mental reactions.

These three are called in Yoga, Shabda (sound), Artha (meaning), and Jnâna (knowledge). In the language of physics and physiology they are called the ethereal vibration, the motion in the nerve and brain, and the mental reaction.

Now these, though distinct processes, have become mixed up in such a fashion as to become quite indistinct. In fact, we cannot now perceive any of these, we only perceive their combined effect, what we call the external object. Every act of perception includes these three, and there is no reason why we should not be able to distinguish them.

*

When, by the previous preparations, it becomes strong and controlled, and has the power of finer perception, the mind should be employed in meditation. This meditation must begin with gross objects and slowly rise to finer and finer, until it becomes objectless.

The mind should first be employed in perceiving the external causes of sensations, then the internal motions, and then its own reaction. When it has succeeded in perceiving the external causes of sensations by themselves, the mind will acquire the power of perceiving all fine material existences, all fine bodies and forms.

When it can succeed in perceiving the motions inside by themselves, it will gain the control of all mental waves, in itself or in others, even before they have translated themselves into physical energy; and when he will be able to perceive the mental reaction by itself, the Yogi will acquire the knowledge of everything, as every sensible object, and every thought is the result of this reaction. Then will he have seen the very foundations of his mind, and it will be under his perfect control.

Different powers will come to the Yogi, and if he yields to the temptations of any one of these, the road to his further progress will be barred. Such is the evil of running after enjoyments. But if he is strong enough to reject even these miraculous powers, he will attain to the goal of Yoga, the complete suppression of the waves in the ocean of the mind.

Then the glory of the soul, undisturbed by the distractions of the mind, or motions of the body, will shine in its full effulgence; and the Yogi will find himself as he is and as he always was, the essence of knowledge, the immortal, the all-pervading.

*

The power of meditation gets us everything. If you want to get power over nature, [you can have it through meditation].

It is through the power of meditation all scientific facts are discovered today. They study the subject and forget everything, their own identity and everything, and then the great fact comes like a flash. Some people think that is inspiration. There is no more inspiration than there is expiration; and never was anything got for nothing.

*

"By constant repetition of the syllable Om and by meditating on its meaning, everything can be obtained"; "All sins are washed away by uttering the name of the Lord"; "He gets all, who resigns himself to the Will of God" — yes, these words of the Shastras and the sages are, no doubt, true.

But, do you see, thousands of us are, for our whole life, meditating on Om, are getting ecstatic in devotion in the name of the Lord, and are crying, "Thy Will be done, I am fully resigned to Thee! " — and what are they actually getting in return? Absolutely nothing!

How do you account for this? The reason lies here, and it must be fully understood.

Whose meditation is real and effective? Who can really resign himself to the Will of God? Who can utter with power irresistible, like that of a thunderbolt, the name of the Lord?

It is he who has earned Chitta-shuddhi, that is, whose mind has been purified by work, or in other words, he who is the Dharmika.

*

When [the mind] is doubtful that is not its great state. Its great state is meditation. It looks upon things and sees things, not identifying itself with anything else. As long as I feel pain, I have identified myself with the body. When I feel joy or pleasure, I have identified myself with the body.

But the high state will look with the same pleasure or blissfulness upon pleasure or upon pain. Every meditation is direct superconsciousness. In perfect concentration the soul becomes actually free from the bonds of the gross body and knows itself as it is.

Whatever one wants, that comes to him. Power and knowledge are already there. The soul identifies itself with that which is powerless matter and thus weeps. It identifies itself with mortal shapes. But if that free soul wants to exercise any power, it will have it.

If it does not, it does not come. He who has known God has become God. There is nothing impossible to such a free soul. No more birth and death for him. He is free for ever.

*

The greatest help to spiritual life is meditation (Dhyâna). In meditation we divest ourselves of all material conditions and feel our divine nature. We do not depend upon any external help in meditation. The touch of the soul can paint the brightest colour even in the dingiest places; it can cast a fragrance over the vilest thing; it can make the wicked divine — and all enmity, all selfishness is effaced.

The less the thought of the body, the better. For it is the body that drags us down. It is attachment, identification, which makes us miserable.

That is the secret: To think that I am the spirit and not the body, and that the whole of this universe with all its relations, with all its good and all its evil, is but as a series of paintings — scenes on a canvas — of which I am the witness.

*

How is it to be attained? In a dozen different ways. Each temperament has its own way. But this is the general principle: get hold of the mind.

The mind is like a lake, and every stone that drops into it raises waves. These waves do not let us see what we are. The full moon is reflected in the water of the lake, but the surface is so disturbed that we do not see the reflection clearly.

Let it be calm. Do not let nature raise the wave. Keep quiet, and then after a little while she will give you up. Then we know what we are.

God is there already, but the mind is so agitated, always running after the senses. You close the senses and [yet] you whirl and whirl about. Just this moment I think I am all right and I will meditate upon God, and then my mind goes to London in one minute. And if I pull it away from there, it goes to New York to think about the things I have done there in the past.

These [waves] are to be stopped by the power of meditation. Slowly and gradually we are to train ourselves. It is no joke — not a question of a day, or years, or maybe of births.

Never mind! The pull must go on. Knowingly, voluntarily, the pull must go on. Inch by inch we will gain ground. We will begin to feel and get real possessions, which no one can take away from us — the wealth that no man can take, the wealth that nobody can destroy, the joy that no misery can hurt any more.

All these years we have depended upon others. If I have a little pleasure and that person goes away, my pleasure is gone. See the folly of man: he depends for happiness upon men! All separations are misery. Naturally. Depending upon wealth for happiness? There is fluctuation of wealth. Depending upon health or upon anything except the unchangeable spirit must bring misery today or tomorrow.

Excepting the infinite spirit, everything else is changing. There is the whirl of change. Permanence is nowhere except in yourself. There is the infinite joy, unchanging.

Meditation is the gate that opens that to us. Prayers, ceremonials, and all the other forms of worship are simply kindergartens of meditation. You pray, you offer something.

A certain theory existed that everything raised one's spiritual power. The use of certain words, flowers, images, temples, ceremonials like the waving of lights brings the mind to that attitude, but that attitude is always in the human soul, nowhere else. [People] are all doing it; but what they do without knowing it, do knowingly.

That is the power of meditation. All knowledge you have — how did it come? From the power of meditation. The soul churned the knowledge out of its own depths.

What knowledge was there ever outside of it? In the long run this power of meditation separates ourselves from the body, and then the soul knows itself as it is — the unborn, the deathless, and birthless being. No more is there any misery, no more births upon this earth, no more evolution. [The soul knows itself as having] ever been perfect and free.

The Power of Meditation

The practice of meditationMeditation has been laid stress upon by all religions. The meditative state of mind is declared by the Yogis to be the highest state in which the mind exists. When the mind is studying the external object, it gets identified with it, loses itself. To use the simile of the old Indian philosopher: the soul of man is like a piece of crystal, but it takes the colour of whatever is near it. Whatever the soul touches it has to take its colour. That is the difficulty. That constitutes the bondage. The colour is so strong, the crystal forgets itself and identifies itself with the colour. Suppose a red flower is near the crystal and the crystal takes the colour and forgets itself, thinks it is red. We have taken the colour of the body and have forgotten what we are. All the difficulties that follow come from that one dead body. All our fears, all worries, anxieties, troubles, mistakes, weakness, evil, are front that one great blunder — that we are bodies. This is the ordinary person. It is the person taking the colour of the flower near to it. We are no more bodies than the crystal is the red flower.

The practice of meditation is pursued. The crystal knows what it is, takes its own colour. It is meditation that brings us nearer to truth than anything else.

*

In India two persons meet. In English they say, "How do you do?" The Indian greeting is, "Are you upon yourself?"

The moment you stand upon something else, you run the risk of being miserable. This is what I mean by meditation — the soul trying to stand upon itself.

That state must surely be the healthiest state of the soul, when it is thinking of itself, residing in its own glory. No, all the other methods that we have — by exciting emotions, prayers, and all that — really have that one end in view. In deep emotional excitement the soul tries to stand upon itself. Although the emotion may arise from anything external, there is concentration of mind.

*

There are three stages in meditation. The first is what is called [Dhâranâ], concentrating the mind upon an object. I try to concentrate my mind upon this glass, excluding every other object from my mind except this glass. But the mind is wavering.

When it has become strong and does not waver so much, it is called [Dhyâna], meditation.

And then there is a still higher state when the differentiation between the glass and myself is lost — [Samâdhi or absorption]. The mind and the glass are identical. I do not see any difference.

All the senses stop and all powers that have been working through other channels of other senses [are focused in the mind]. Then this glass is under the power of the mind entirely. This is to be realised. It is a tremendous play played by the Yogis.

*

Take for granted, the external object exists. Then that which is really outside of us is not what we see. The glass that I see is not the external object certainly. That external something which is the glass I do not know and will never know.

Something produces an impression upon me. Immediately I send the reaction towards that, and the glass is the result of the combination of these two. Action from outside — X. Action from inside — Y. The glass is XY.

When you look at X, call it external world — at Y, internal world If you try to distinguish which is your mind and which is the world — there is no such distinction. The world is the combination of you and something else.

Let us take another example. You are dropping stones upon the smooth surface of a lake. Every stone you drop is followed by a reaction. The stone is covered by the little waves in the lake.

Similarly, external things are like the stones dropping into the lake of the mind. So we do not really see the external . . .; we see the wave only.

These waves that rise in the mind have caused many things outside. We are not discussing the [merits of] idealism and realism. We take for granted that things exist outside, but what we see is different from things that exist outside, as we see what exists outside plus ourselves.

Suppose I take my contribution out of the glass. What remains? Almost nothing. The glass will disappear.

If I take my contribution from the table, what would remain of the table? Certainly not this table, because it was a mixture of the outside plus my contribution. The poor lake has got to throw the wave towards the stone whenever [the stone] is thrown in it. The mind must create the wave towards any sensation.

Suppose we can withhold the mind. At once we are masters. We refuse to contribute our share to all these phenomena. If I do not contribute my share, it has got to stop.

*

You are creating this bondage all the time. How? By putting in your share. We are all making our own beds, forging our own chains.

When the identifying ceases between this external object and myself, then I will be able to take my contribution off, and this thing will disappear. Then I will say, “Here is the glass”, and then take my mind off, and it disappears.

If you can take away your share, you can walk upon water. Why should it drown you any more? What of poison? No more difficulties. In every phenomenon in nature you contribute at least half, and nature brings half. If your half is taken off, the thing must stop.

To every action there is equal reaction. If a man strikes me and wounds me it is that man’s actions and my body’s reaction. Suppose I have so much power over the body that I can resist even that automatic action.

Can such power be attained? The books say it can. If you stumble on [it], it is a miracle. If you learn it scientifically, it is Yoga.

I have seen people healed by the power of mind. There is the miracle worker. We say he prays and the man is healed. Another man says, "Not at all. It is just the power of the mind. The man is scientific. He knows what he is about."

*

The power of meditation gets us everything. If you want to get power over nature, [you can have it through meditation]. It is through the power of meditation all scientific facts are discovered today. They study the subject and forget everything, their own identity and everything, and then the great fact comes like a flash. Some people think that is inspiration. There is no more inspiration than there is expiration; and never was anything got for nothing.

The highest so-called inspiration was the work of Jesus. He worked hard for ages in previous births. That was the result of his previous work — hard work. It is all nonsense to talk about inspiration. Had it been, it would have fallen like rain.

Inspired people in any line of thought only come among nations who have general education and [culture]. There is no inspiration. Whatever passes for inspiration is the result that comes from causes already in the mind. One day, flash comes the result! Their past work was the [cause].

Therein also you see the power of meditation — intensity of thought. These men churn up their own souls. Great truths come to the surface and become manifest.

Therefore the practice of meditation is the great scientific method of knowledge. There is no knowledge without the power of meditation. From ignorance, superstition, etc. we can get cured by meditation for the time being and no more.

[Suppose] a man has told me that if you drink such a poison you will be killed, and another man comes in the night and says, "Go drink the poison!" and I am not killed, [what happens is this:] my mind cut out from the meditation the identity between the poison and myself just for the time being. In another case of [drinking] the poison, I will be killed.

If I know the reason and scientifically raise myself up to that [state of meditation], I can save anyone. That is what the books say; but how far it is correct you must appraise.

*

I am asked, "Why do you Indian people not conquer these things? You claim all the time to be superior to all other people. You practice Yoga and do it quicker than anybody else. You are fitter. Carry it out! If you are a great people, you ought to have a great system. You will have to say good-bye to all the gods. Let them go to sleep as you take up the great philosophers.

"You are mere babies, as superstitious as the rest of the world. And all your claims are failures. If you have the claims, stand up and be bold, and all the heaven that ever existed is yours. There is the musk deer with fragrance inside, and he does not know where the fragrance [comes from]. Then after days and days he finds it in himself. All these gods and demons are within them. Find out, by the powers of reason, education, and culture that it is all in yourself. No more gods and superstitions. You want to be rational, to be Yogis, really spiritual."

[My reply is: With you too] everything is material. What is more material than God sitting on a throne? You look down upon the poor man who is worshipping the image. You are no better.

And you, gold worshippers, what are you? The image worshipper worships his god, something that he can see. But you do not even do that. You do not worship the spirit nor something that you can understand.

Word worshippers! "God is spirit!" God is spirit and should be worshipped in spirit and faith. Where does the spirit reside? On a tree? On a cloud?

What do you mean by God being ours? You are the spirit. That is the first fundamental belief you must never give up. I am the spiritual being. It is there. All this skill of Yoga and this system of meditation and everything is just to find Him there.

*

Why am I saying all this just now? Until you fix the location, you cannot talk. You fix it up in heaven and all the world ever except in the right place. I am spirit, and therefore the spirit of all spirits must be in my soul. Those who think it anywhere else are ignorant.

Therefore it is to be sought here in this heaven; all the heaven that ever existed [is within myself]. There are some sages who, knowing this, turn their eyes inward and find the spirit of all spirits in their own spirit. That is the scope of meditation. Find out the truth about God and about your own soul and thus attain to liberation.

You are all running after life, and we find that is foolishness. There is something much higher than life even. This life is inferior, material. Why should I live at all? I am something higher than life. Living is always slavery. We always get mixed up. Everything is a continuous chain of slavery.

You get something, and no man can teach another. It is through experience [we learn]. That young man cannot be persuaded that there are any difficulties in life. You cannot persuade the old man that life is all smooth. He has had many experiences. That is the difference.

By the power of meditation we have got to control, step by step, all these things. We have seen philosophically that all these differentiations — spirit, mind, matter, etc. — [have no real existences. Whatever exists is one. There cannot be many.

That is what is meant by science and knowledge. Ignorance sees manifold. Knowledge realises one. Reducing the many into one is science. The whole of the universe has been demonstrated into one. That science is called the science of Vedanta. The whole universe is one. The one runs through all this seeming variety.

We have all these variations now and we see them — what we call the five elements: solid, liquid, gaseous, luminous, ethereal. After that the state of existence is mental and beyond that spiritual.

Not that spirit is one and mind is another, ether another, and so on. It is the one existence appearing in all these variations. To go back, the solid must become liquid. The way [the elements evolved] they must go back. The solids will become liquid, etherised. This is the idea of the macrocosm — and universal. There is the external universe and universal spirit, mind, ether, gas, luminosity, liquid, solid.

The same with the mind. I am just exactly the same in the microcosm. I am the spirit; I am mind; I am the ether, solid, liquid, gas. What I want to do is to go back to my spiritual state. It is for the individual to live the life of the universe in one short life. Thus man can be free in this life. He in his own short lifetime shall have the power to live the whole extent of life.

We all struggle. If we cannot reach the Absolute, we will get somewhere, and it will be better than we are now.

Meditation consists in this practice [of dissolving every thing into the ultimate Reality — spirit]. The solid melts into liquid, that into gas, gas into ether, then mind, and mind will melt away. All is spirit.

Some of the Yogis claim that this body will become liquid etc. You will be able to do any thing with it — make it little, or gas pass through this wall — they claim. I do not know. I have never seen anybody do it. But it is in the books. We have no reason to disbelieve the books.

Possibly, some of us will be able to do it in this life. Like a flash it comes, as the result of our past work. Who knows but some here are old Yogis with just a little to do to finish the whole work. Practice!

Meditation, you know, comes by a process imagination. You go through all these processes purification of the elements — making the one melt the other, that into the next higher, that into mind, that into spirit, and then you are spirit. [14]

Spirit is always free, omnipotent, omniscient. Of course, under God. There cannot be many Gods. These liberated souls are wonderfully powerful, almost omnipotent. [But] none can be as powerful as God. If one [liberated soul] said, "I will make this planet go this way", and another said, "I will make it go that way", [there would be confusion].

Don't you make this mistake! When I say in English, "I am God!" it is because I have no better word. In Sanskrit, God means absolute existence, knowledge, and wisdom, infinite self-luminous consciousness. No person. It is impersonal.

I am never Râma [never one with Ishvara, the personal aspect of God], but I am [one with Brahman, the impersonal, all-pervading existence].

Here is a huge mass of clay. Out of that clay I made a little [mouse] and you made a little [elephant]. Both are clay. Melt both down. They are essentially one. "I and my Father are one." [But the clay mouse can never be one with the clay elephant.]

I stop somewhere; I have a little knowledge. You a little more; you stop somewhere. There is one soul which is the greatest of all. This is Ishvara, Lord of Yoga [God as Creator, with attributes]. He is the individual. He is omnipotent. He resides in every heart. There is no body. He does not need a body. All you get by the practice of meditation etc., you can get by meditation upon Ishvara, Lord of Yogis.

*

Thousands of divine beings are standing about you. You do not see them because our world is determined by our senses. We can only see this outside. Let us call it X. We see that X according to our mental state.

Let us take the tree standing outside. A thief came and what did he see in the stump? A policeman. The child saw a huge ghost. The young man was waiting for his sweetheart, and what did he see? His sweetheart.

But the stump of the tree had not changed. It remained the same. This is God Himself, and with our foolishness we see Him to be man, to be dust, to be dumb, miserable.

Those who are similarly constituted will group together naturally and live in the same world. Otherwise stated, you live in the same place. All the heavens and all the hells are right here.

For example: [take planes in the form of] big circles cutting each other at certain points. On this plane in one circle we can be in touch with a certain point in another [circle]. If the mind gets to the centre, you begin to be conscious on all planes.

In meditation sometimes you touch another plane, and you see other beings, disembodied spirits, and so on. You get there by the power of meditation. This power is changing our senses, you see, refining our senses.

If you begin to practise meditation five days, you will feel the pain from within these centres [of conciousness] and hearing [becomes finer]. That is why all the Indian gods have three eyes. That is the psychic eye that opens out and shows you spiritual things.

As this power of Kundalini rises from one centre to the other in the spine, it changes the senses and you begin to see this world another. It is heaven. You cannot talk.

Then the Kundalini goes down to the lower centres. You are again man until the Kundalini reaches the brain, all the centres have been passed, and the whole vision vanishes and you [perceive] nothing but the one existence. You are God. All heavens you make out of Him, all worlds out of Him. He is the one existence. Nothing else exists.

Meditation has been laid stress upon by all religions. The meditative state of mind is declared by the Yogis to be the highest state in which the mind exists. When the mind is studying the external object, it gets identified with it, loses itself. To use the simile of the old Indian philosopher: the soul of man is like a piece of crystal, but it takes the colour of whatever is near it. Whatever the soul touches ... it has to take its colour. That is the difficulty. That constitutes the bondage. The colour is so strong, the crystal forgets itself and identifies itself with the colour. Suppose a red flower is near the crystal and the crystal takes the colour and forgets itself, thinks it is red. We have taken the colour of the body and have forgotten what we are. All the difficulties that follow come from that one dead body. All our fears, all worries, anxieties, troubles, mistakes, weakness, evil, are front that one great blunder — that we are bodies. This is the ordinary person. It is the person taking the colour of the flower near to it. We are no more bodies than the crystal is the red flower.

The practice of meditation is pursued. The crystal knows what it is, takes its own colour. It is meditation that brings us nearer to truth than anything else. ...

In India two persons meet. In English they say, "How do you do?" The Indian greeting is, "Are you upon yourself?" The moment you stand upon something else, you run the risk of being miserable. This is what I mean by meditation — the soul trying to stand upon itself. That state must surely be the healthiest state of the soul, when it is thinking of itself, residing in its own glory. No, all the other methods that we have — by exciting emotions, prayers, and all that — really have that one end in view. In deep emotional excitement the soul tries to stand upon itself. Although the emotion may arise from anything external, there is concentration of mind.

There are three stages in meditation. The first is what is called [Dhâranâ], concentrating the mind upon an object. I try to concentrate my mind upon this glass, excluding every other object from my mind except this glass. But the mind is wavering . . . When it has become strong and does not waver so much, it is called [Dhyâna], meditation. And then there is a still higher state when the differentiation between the glass and myself is lost — [Samâdhi or absorption]. The mind and the glass are identical. I do not see any difference. All the senses stop and all powers that have been working through other channels of other senses [are focused in the mind]. Then this glass is under the power of the mind entirely. This is to be realised. It is a tremendous play played by the Yogis. ... Take for granted, the external object exists. Then that which is really outside of us is not what we see. The glass that I see is not the external object certainly. That external something which is the glass I do not know and will never know.

Something produces an impression upon me. Immediately I send the reaction towards that, and the glass is the result of the combination of these two. Action from outside — X. Action from inside — Y. The glass is XY. When you look at X, call it external world — at Y, internal world . . . If you try to distinguish which is your mind and which is the world — there is no such distinction. The world is the combination of you and something else. ...

Let us take another example. You are dropping stones upon the smooth surface of a lake. Every stone you drop is followed by a reaction. The stone is covered by the little waves in the lake. Similarly, external things are like the stones dropping into the lake of the mind. So we do not really see the external . . .; we see the wave only. . . .

These waves that rise in the mind have caused many things outside. We are not discussing the [merits of] idealism and realism. We take for granted that things exist outside, but what we see is different from things that exist outside, as we see what exists outside plus ourselves.

Suppose I take my contribution out of the glass. What remains? Almost nothing. The glass will disappear. If I take my contribution from the table, what would remain of the table? Certainly not this table, because it was a mixture of the outside plus my contribution. The poor lake has got to throw the wave towards the stone whenever [the stone] is thrown in it. The mind must create the wave towards any sensation. Suppose . . . we can withhold the mind. At once we are masters. We refuse to contribute our share to all these phenomena.... If I do not contribute my share, it has got to stop.

You are creating this bondage all the time. How? By putting in your share. We are all making our own beds, forging our own chains.... When the identifying ceases between this external object and myself, then I will be able to take my contribution off, and this thing will disappear. Then I will say, "Here is the glass", and then take my mind off, and it disappears.... If you can take away your share, you can walk upon water. Why should it drown you any more? What of poison? No more difficulties. In every phenomenon in nature you contribute at least half, and nature brings half. If your half is taken off, the thing must stop.

... To every action there is equal reaction.... If a man strikes me and wounds me it is that man's actions and my body's reaction. ... Suppose I have so much power over the body that I can resist even that automatic action. Can such power be attained? The books say it can. ... If you stumble on [it], it is a miracle. If you learn it scientifically, it is Yoga.

I have seen people healed by the power of mind. There is the miracle worker. We say he prays and the man is healed. Another man says, "Not at all. It is just the power of the mind. The man is scientific. He knows what he is about."

The power of meditation gets us everything. If you want to get power over nature, [you can have it through meditation]. It is through the power of meditation all scientific facts are discovered today. They study the subject and forget everything, their own identity and everything, and then the great fact comes like a flash. Some people think that is inspiration. There is no more inspiration than there is expiration; and never was anything got for nothing.

The highest so-called inspiration was the work of Jesus. He worked hard for ages in previous births. That was the result of his previous work — hard work. ... It is all nonsense to talk about inspiration. Had it been, it would have fallen like rain. Inspired people in any line of thought only come among nations who have general education and [culture]. There is no inspiration. . . . Whatever passes for inspiration is the result that comes from causes already in the mind. One day, flash comes the result! Their past work was the [cause].

Therein also you see the power of meditation — intensity of thought. These men churn up their own souls. Great truths come to the surface and become manifest. Therefore the practice of meditation is the great scientific method of knowledge. There is no knowledge without the power of meditation. From ignorance, superstition, etc. we can get cured by meditation for the time being and no more. [Suppose] a man has told me that if you drink such a poison you will be killed, and another man comes in the night and says, "Go drink the poison!" and I am not killed, [what happens is this:] my mind cut out from the meditation the identity between the poison and myself just for the time being. In another case of [drinking] the poison, I will be killed.

If I know the reason and scientifically raise myself up to that [state of meditation], I can save anyone. That is what the books say; but how far it is correct you must appraise.

I am asked, "Why do you Indian people not conquer these things? You claim all the time to be superior to all other people. You practice Yoga and do it quicker than anybody else. You are fitter. Carry it out! If you are a great people, you ought to have a great system. You will have to say good-bye to all the gods. Let them go to sleep as you take up the great philosophers. You are mere babies, as superstitious as the rest of the world. And all your claims are failures. If you have the claims, stand up and be bold, and all the heaven that ever existed is yours. There is the musk deer with fragrance inside, and he does not know where the fragrance [comes from]. Then after days and days he finds it in himself. All these gods and demons are within them. Find out, by the powers of reason, education, and culture that it is all in yourself. No more gods and superstitions. You want to be rational, to be Yogis, really spiritual."

[My reply is: With you too] everything is material What is more material than God sitting on a throne? You look down upon the poor man who is worshipping the image. You are no better. And you, gold worshippers, what are you? The image worshipper worships his god, something that he can see. But you do not even do that. You do not worship the spirit nor something that you can understand. ... Word worshippers! "God is spirit!" God is spirit and should be worshipped in spirit and faith. Where does the spirit reside? On a tree? On a cloud? What do you mean by God being ours ? You are the spirit. That is the first fundamental belief you must never give up. I am the spiritual being. It is there. All this skill of Yoga and this system of meditation and everything is just to find Him there.

Why am I saying all this just now? Until you fix the location, you cannot talk. You fix it up in heaven and all the world ever except in the right place. I am spirit, and therefore the spirit of all spirits must be in my soul. Those who think it anywhere else are ignorant. Therefore it is to be sought here in this heaven; all the heaven that ever existed [is within myself]. There are some sages who, knowing this, turn their eyes inward and find the spirit of all spirits in their own spirit. That is the scope of meditation. Find out the truth about God and about your own soul and thus attain to liberation. ...

You are all running after life, and we find that is foolishness. There is something much higher than life even. This life is inferior, material. Why should I live at all? I am something higher than life. Living is always slavery. We always get mixed up. ... Everything is a continuous chain of slavery.

You get something, and no man can teach another. It is through experience [we learn]. ... That young man cannot be persuaded that there are any difficulties in life. You cannot persuade the old man that life is all smooth. He has had many experiences. That is the difference.

By the power of meditation we have got to control, step by step, all these things.

We have seen philosophically that all these differentiations — spirit, mind, matter, etc. — [have no real existences. ... Whatever exists is one. There cannot be many. That is what is meant by science and knowledge. Ignorance sees manifold. Knowledge realises one. ... Reducing the many into one is science. ... The whole of the universe has been demonstrated into one. That science is called the science of Vedanta. The whole universe is one. The one runs through all this seeming variety. ...

We have all these variations now and we see them — what we call the five elements: solid, liquid, gaseous, luminous, ethereal. After that the state of existence is mental and beyond that spiritual. Not that spirit is one and mind is another, ether another, and so on. It is the one existence appearing in all these variations. To go back, the solid must become liquid. The way [the elements evolved] they must go back. The solids will become liquid, etherised. This is the idea of the macrocosm — and universal. There is the external universe and universal spirit, mind, ether, gas, luminosity, liquid, solid.

The same with the mind. I am just exactly the same in the microcosm. I am the spirit; I am mind; I am the ether, solid, liquid, gas. What I want to do is to go back to my spiritual state. It is for the individual to live the life of the universe in one short life. Thus man can be free in this life. He in his own short lifetime shall have the power to live the whole extent of life....

We all struggle. . . . If we cannot reach the Absolute, we will get somewhere, and it will be better than we are now.

Meditation consists in this practice [of dissolving every thing into the ultimate Reality — spirit]. The solid melts into liquid, that into gas, gas into ether, then mind, and mind will melt away. All is spirit.

Some of the Yogis claim that this body will become liquid etc. You will be able to do any thing with it — make it little, or gas pass through this wall — they claim. I do not know. I have never seen anybody do it. But it is in the books. We have no reason to disbelieve the books.

Possibly, some of us will be able to do it in this life. Like a flash it comes, as the result of our past work. Who knows but some here are old Yogis with just a little to do to finish the whole work. Practice!

Meditation, you know, comes by a process imagination. You go through all these processes purification of the elements — making the one melt the other, that into the next higher, that into mind, that into spirit, and then you are spirit. [14]

Spirit is always free, omnipotent, omniscient. Of course, under God. There cannot be many Gods. These liberated souls are wonderfully powerful, almost omnipotent. [But] none can be as powerful as God. If one [liberated soul] said, "I will make this planet go this way", and another said, "I will make it go that way", [there would be confusion].

Don't you make this mistake! When I say in English, "I am God!" it is because I have no better word. In Sanskrit, God means absolute existence, knowledge, and wisdom, infinite self-luminous consciousness. No person. It is impersonal. ...

I am never Râma [never one with Ishvara, the personal aspect of God], but I am [one with Brahman, the impersonal, all-pervading existence]. Here is a huge mass of clay. Out of that clay I made a little [mouse] and you made a little [elephant]. Both are clay. Melt both down They are essentially one. "I and my Father are one." [But the clay mouse can never be one with the clay elephant.]

I stop somewhere; I have a little knowledge. You a little more; you stop somewhere. There is one soul which is the greatest of all. This is Ishvara, Lord of Yoga [God as Creator, with attributes]. He is the individual. He is omnipotent. He resides in every heart. There is no body. He does not need a body. All you get by the practice of meditation etc., you can get by meditation upon Ishvara, Lord of Yogis. ...

The same can be attained by meditating upon a great soul; or upon the harmony of life. These are called objective meditations. So you begin to meditate upon certain external things, objective things, either outside or inside. If you take a long sentence, that is no meditation at all. That is simply trying to get the mind collected by repetition. Meditation means the mind is turned back upon itself. The mind stops all the [thought-waves] and the world stops. Your consciousness expands. Every time you meditate you will keep your growth. ... Work a little harder, more and more, and meditation comes. You do not feel the body or anything else. When you come out of it after the hour, you have had the most beautiful rest you ever had in your life. That is the only way you ever give rest to your system. Not even the deepest sleep will give you such rest as that. The mind goes on jumping even in deepest sleep. Just those few minutes [in meditation] your brain has almost stopped. Just a little vitality is kept up. You forget the body. You may be cut to pieces and not feel it at all. You feel such pleasure in it. You become so light. This perfect rest we will get in meditation.

Then, meditation upon different objects. There are meditations upon different centres of the spine. [According to the Yogis, there are two nerves in the spinal column, called Idâ and Pingalâ.They are the main channels through which the afferent and efferent currents travel.] The hollow [canal called Sushumnâ] runs through the middle of the spinal column. The Yogis claim this cord is closed, but by the power of meditation it has to be opened. The energy has to be sent down to [the base of the spine], and the Kundalini rises. The world will be changed. ... (See Complete Works , Vol. I, The Psychic Prana)

Thousands of divine beings are standing about you. You do not see them because our world is determined by our senses. We can only see this outside. Let us call it X. We see that X according to our mental state. Let us take the tree standing outside. A thief came and what did he see in the stump? A policeman. The child saw a huge ghost. The young man was waiting for his sweetheart, and what did he see? His sweetheart. But the stump of the tree had not changed. It remained the same. This is God Himself, and with our foolishness we see Him to be man, to be dust, to be dumb, miserable.

Those who are similarly constituted will group together naturally and live in the same world. Otherwise stated, you live in the same place. All the heavens and all the hells are right here. For example: [take planes in the form of] big circles cutting each other at certain points. . . . On this plane in one circle we can be in touch with a certain point in another [circle]. If the mind gets to the centre, you begin to be conscious on all planes. In meditation sometimes you touch another plane, and you see other beings, disembodied spirits, and so on. You get there by the power of meditation. This power is changing our senses, you see, refining our senses. If you begin to practise meditation five days, you will feel the pain from within these centres [of conciousness] and hearing [becomes finer]. ... (See Complete Works , Vol. I, Pratyahara and Dharana). That is why all the Indian gods have three eyes. That is the psychic eye that opens out and shows you spiritual things.

As this power of Kundalini rises from one centre to the other in the spine, it changes the senses and you begin to see this world another. It is heaven. You cannot talk. Then the Kundalini goes down to the lower centres. You are again man until the Kundalini reaches the brain, all the centres have been passed, and the whole vision vanishes and you [perceive] . . . nothing but the one existence. You are God. All heavens you make out of Him, all worlds out of Him. He is the one existence. Nothing else exists.

The Practice of Meditation

Yoga has essentially to do with the meditative side of religion, rather than the ethical side, though, of necessity, a little of the latter has to be considered. Men and women are growing to desire more than mere revelation, so called. They want facts in their own consciousness.

Only through experience can there be any reality in religion. Spiritual facts are to be gathered mostly from the superconscious state of mind.

Let us put ourselves into the same condition as did those who claim to have had special experiences; then if we have similar experiences, they become facts for us. We can see all that another has seen; a thing that happened once can happen again, nay, must, under the same circumstances.

Raja-Yoga teaches us how to reach the superconscious state. All the great religions recognise this state in some form; but in India, special attention is paid to this side of religion.

In the beginning, some mechanical means may help us to acquire this state; but mechanical means alone can never accomplish much. Certain positions, certain modes of breathing, help to harmonise and concentrate the mind, but with these must go purity and strong desire for God, or realisation.

The attempt to sit down and fix the mind on one idea and hold it there will prove to most people that there is some need for help to enable them to do this successfully. The mind has to be gradually and systematically brought under control. The will has to be strengthened by slow, continuous, and persevering drill.

This is no child's play, no fad to be tried one day and discarded the next. It is a life's work; and the end to be attained is well worth all that it can cost us to reach it; being nothing less than the realisation of our absolute oneness with the Divine. Surely, with this end in view, and with the knowledge that we can certainly succeed, no price can be too great to pay.

*

No amount of reasoning which I can give you will be proof to you, until you have demonstrated it for yourselves. As soon as you begin to feel these currents in motion all over you, doubts will vanish, but it requires hard practice every day.

You must practice at least twice every day, and the best times are towards the morning and the evening. When night passes into day, and day into night, a state of relative calmness ensues. The early morning and the early evening are the two periods of calmness.

Your body will have a like tendency to become calm at those times. We should take advantage of that natural condition and begin then to practice. Make it a rule not to eat until you have practiced; if you do this, the sheer force of hunger will break your laziness.

In India they teach children never to eat until they have practiced or worshipped, and it becomes natural to them after a time; a boy will not feel hungry until he has bathed and practiced.

Sit in a straight posture, and the first thing to do is to send a current of holy thought to all creation. Mentally repeat, "Let all beings be happy; let all beings be peaceful; let all beings be blissful." So do to the east, south, north and west.

The more you do that the better you will feel yourself. You will find at last that the easiest way to make ourselves healthy is to see that others are healthy, and the easiest way to make ourselves happy is to see that others are happy.

After doing that, those who believe in God should pray — not for money, not for health, nor for heaven; pray for knowledge and light; every other prayer is selfish.

Then the next thing to do is to think of your own body, and see that it is strong and healthy; it is the best instrument you have. Think of it as being as strong as adamant, and that with the help of this body you will cross the ocean of life.

Freedom is never to be reached by the weak. Throw away all weakness. Tell your body that it is strong, tell your mind that it is strong, and have unbounded faith and hope in yourself.

*

The greater part of the practical lessons which the Yogi gives us is in the mind, the power of concentration and meditation. We have become so materialistic. When we think of ourselves, we find only the body. The body has become the ideal, nothing else. Therefore a little physical help is necessary.

First, to sit in the posture in which you can sit still for a long time. All the nerve currents which are working pass along the spine. The spine is not intended to support the weight of the body.

Therefore the posture must be such that the weight of the body is not on the spine. Let it be free from all pressure.

*

There are some other preliminary things. There is the great question of food and exercise.

The food must be simple and taken several times [a day] instead of once or twice. Never get very hungry. "He who eats too much cannot be a Yogi. He who fasts too much cannot be a Yogi. He who sleeps too much cannot be a Yogi, nor he who keeps awake too much." (Gita, VI. 16.)

He who does not do any work and he who works too hard cannot succeed. Proper food, proper exercise, proper sleep, proper wakefulness — these are necessary for any success.

What the proper food is, what kind, we have to determine ourselves. Nobody can determine that [for us].

As a general practice, we have to shun exciting food. We do not know how to vary our diet with our occupation. We always forget that it is the food out of which we manufacture everything we have. So the amount and kind of energy that we want, the food must determine.

Violent exercises are not all necessary. If you want to be muscular, Yoga is not for you. You have to manufacture a finer organism than you have now.

Violent exercises are positively hurtful. Live amongst those who do not take too much exercise. If you do not take violent exercise, you will live longer. You do not want to burn out your lamp in muscles! People who work with their brains are the longest-lived people.

Do not burn the lamp quickly. Let it burn slowly and gently. Every anxiety, every violent exercise — physical and mental — [means] you are burning the lamp.

The proper diet means, generally, simply do not eat highly spiced foods. There are three sorts of mind, says the Yogi, according to the elements of nature. One is the dull mind, which covers the luminosity of the soul. Then there is that which makes people active, and lastly, that which makes them calm and peaceful.

Now there are persons born with the tendency to sleep all the time. Their taste will be towards that type of food which is rotting — crawling cheese. They will eat cheese that fairly jumps off the table. It is a natural tendency with them.

Then active people. Their taste is for everything hot and pungent, strong alcohol.

Sâttvika people are very thoughtful, quiet, and patient. They take food in small quantities, and never anything bad.

*

"He who hates none, who is the friend of all, who is merciful to all, who has nothing of his own, who is free from egoism, who is even-minded in pain and pleasure, who is forbearing, who is always satisfied, who works always in Yoga, whose self has become controlled, whose will is firm, whose mind and intellect are given up unto Me, such a one is My beloved Bhakta.

"From whom comes no disturbance, who cannot be disturbed by others, who is free from joy, anger, fear, and anxiety, such a one is My beloved.

"He who does not depend on anything, who is pure and active, who does not care whether good comes or evil, and never becomes miserable, who has given up all efforts for himself; who is the same in praise or in blame, with a silent, thoughtful mind, blessed with what little comes in his way, homeless, for the whole world is his home, and who is steady in his ideas, such a one is My beloved Bhakta."

Such alone become Yogis.

*

Meditate every day alone. Everything will open up of itself. Now the Divine Mother — the embodiment of illumination — is sleeping within, hence you do not understand this. She is the Kundalini.

When, before meditating, you proceed to "purify the nerves", you must mentally strike hard on the Kundalini in the Muladhara (sacral plexus), and repeat, "Arise, Mother, arise!" One must practise these slowly.

During meditation, suppress the emotional side altogether. This is a great source of danger. Those that are very emotional no doubt have their Kundalini rushing quickly upwards, but it is as quick to come down as to go up. And when it does come down, it leaves the devotee in a state of utter ruin.

It is for this reason that Kirtanas and other auxiliaries to emotional development have a great drawback. It is true that by dancing and jumping, etc. through a momentary impulse, that power is made to course upwards, but it is never enduring. On the contrary when it traces back its course, it rouses violent lust in the individual.

Listening to my lectures in America, through temporary excitement many among the audience used to get into an ecstatic state, and some would even become motionless like statues. But on inquiry I afterwards found that many of them had an excess of the carnal instinct immediately after that state. But this happens simply owing to a lack of steady practice in meditation and concentration.

*

You yourself will be the object of your meditation. Think and meditate that you are the omnipresent Atman. "I am neither the body, nor the mind, nor the Buddhi (determinative faculty), neither the gross nor the subtle body"– by this process of elimination, immerse your mind in the transcendent knowledge which is your real nature.

Kill the mind by thus plunging it repeatedly in this. Then only you will realise the Essence of Intelligence, or be established in your real nature. Knower and known, meditator and the object meditated upon will then become one, and the cessation of all phenomenal superimpositions will follow.

This is styled in the Shastras as the transcendence of the triad or relative knowledge (Triputibheda). There is no relative or conditioned knowledge in this state. When the Atman is the only knower, by what means can you possibly know It? The Atman is Knowledge, the Atman is Intelligence, the Atman is Sachchidananda.

It is through the inscrutable power of Maya, which cannot be indicated as either existent or non – existent, that the relative consciousness has come upon the Jiva who is none other than Brahman. This is generally known as the conscious state.

And the state in which this duality of relative existence becomes one in the pure Brahman is called in the scriptures the superconscious state and described in such words as, "it is like an ocean perfectly at rest and without a name" (Vivekachudamani, 410).

*

There is another way in which this idea of mercy and selfless charity can be put into practice; that is, by looking upon work as "worship" in case we believe in a Personal God. Here we give up all the fruits our work unto the Lord, and worshipping Him thus, we have no right to expect anything from mankind for the work we do.

The Lord Himself works incessantly and is ever without attachment. Just as water cannot wet the lotus leaf, so work cannot bind the unselfish man by giving rise to attachment to results. The selfless and unattached man may live in the very heart of a crowded and sinful city; he will not be touched by sin.

*

This idea of complete self-sacrifice is illustrated in the following story: After the battle of Kurukshetra the five Pândava brothers performed a great sacrifice and made very large gifts to the poor. All people expressed amazement at the greatness and richness of the sacrifice, and said that such a sacrifice the world had never seen before.

But, after the ceremony, there came a little mongoose, half of whose body was golden, and the other half brown; and he began to roll on the floor of the sacrificial hall. He said to those around, "You are all liars; this is no sacrifice."

"What!" they exclaimed, "you say this is no sacrifice; do you not know how money and jewels were poured out to the poor and every one became rich and happy? This was the most wonderful sacrifice any man ever performed."

But the mongoose said, "There was once a little village, and in it there dwelt a poor Brahmin with his wife, his son, and his son's wife. They were very poor and lived on small gifts made to them for preaching and teaching. There came in that land a three years' famine, and the poor Brahmin suffered more than ever. At last when the family had starved for days, the father brought home one morning a little barley flour, which he had been fortunate enough to obtain, and he divided it into four parts, one for each member of the family. They prepared it for their meal, and just as they were about to eat, there was a knock at the door. The father opened it, and there stood a guest. Now in India a guest is a sacred person; he is as a god for the time being, and must be treated as such. So the poor Brahmin said, 'Come in, sir; you are welcome,' He set before the guest his own portion of the food, which the guest quickly ate and said, 'Oh, sir, you have killed me; I have been starving for ten days, and this little bit has but increased my hunger.' Then the wife said to her husband, 'Give him my share,' but the husband said, 'Not so.' The wife however insisted, saying, 'Here is a poor man, and it is our duty as householders to see that he is fed, and it is my duty as a wife to give him my portion, seeing that you have no more to offer him.' Then she gave her share to the guest, which he ate, and said he was still burning with hunger. So the son said, 'Take my portion also; it is the duty of a son to help his father to fulfil his obligations.' The guest ate that, but remained still unsatisfied; so the son's wife gave him her portion also. That was sufficient, and the guest departed, blessing them. That night those four people died of starvation. A few granules of that flour had fallen on the floor; and when I rolled my body on them, half of it became golden, as you see. Since then I have been travelling all over the world, hoping to find another sacrifice like that, but nowhere have I found one; nowhere else has the other half of my body been turned into gold.

That is why I say this is no sacrifice."

*

We are all struggling day and night to get rid of misery. We cannot do it by work. Work will produce more work. It is only possible if there is someone who is free himself and lends us a hand. "Hear, ye children of immortality, all those that reside in this plane and all those that reside in the heavens above, I have found the secret", says the great sage. "I have found Him who is beyond all darkness. Through His mercy alone we cross this ocean of life."

*

Think of a space in your heart, and in the midst of that space think that a flame is burning. Think of that flame as your own soul and inside the flame is another effulgent light, and that is the Soul of your soul, God. Meditate upon that in the heart.

Chastity, non-injury, forgiving even the greatest enemy, truth, faith in the Lord, these are all different Vrittis. Be not afraid if you are not perfect in all of these; work, they will come.

He who has given up all attachment, all fear, and all anger, he whose whole soul has gone unto the Lord, he who has taken refuge in the Lord, whose heart has become purified, with whatsoever desire he comes to the Lord, He will grant that to him. Therefore, worship Him through knowledge, love, or renunciation.

Religion As a Practice

We read many books, many scriptures. We get various ideas from our childhood, and change them every now and then. We understand what is meant by theoretical religion. We think we understand what is meant by practical religion. Now I am going to present to you my idea of practical religion.

We hear all around us about practical religion, and analysing all that, we find that it can be brought down to one conception — charity to our fellow beings. Is that all of religion? Every day we hear in this country about practical Christianity — that a man has done some good to his fellow beings. Is that all?

What is the goal of life? Is this world the goal of life? Nothing more? Are we to be just what we are, nothing more? Is man to be a machine which runs smoothly without a hitch anywhere? Are all the sufferings he experiences today all he can have, and doesn't he want anything more?

The highest dream of many religions is the world. The vast majority of people are dreaming of the time when there will be no more disease, sickness, poverty, or misery of any kind. They will have a good time all around. Practical religion, therefore, simply means. "Clean the streets! Make it nice!" We see how all enjoy it.

Is enjoyment the goal of life? Were it so, it would be a tremendous mistake to become a man at all. What man can enjoy a meal with more gusto than the dog or the cat? Go to a menagerie and see the [wild animals] tearing the flesh from the bone. Go back and become a bird! What a mistake then to become a man! Vain have been my years — hundreds of years — of struggle only to become the man of sense-enjoyments.

*

Mark, therefore, the ordinary theory of practical religion, what it leads to. Charity is great, but the moment you say it is all, you run the risk of running into materialism. It is not religion. It is no better than atheism - a little less.

You Christians, have you found nothing else in the Bible than working for fellow creatures, building hospitals? Here stands a shopkeeper and says how Jesus would have kept the shop! Jesus would neither have kept a saloon, nor a shop, nor have edited a newspaper. That sort of practical religion is good, not bad; but it is just kindergarten religion. It leads nowhere.

If you believe in God, if you are Christians and repeat everyday, "Thy will be done", just think what it means! You say every moment, "Thy will be done", really meaning, "My will be done by Thee, O God." The Infinite is working His own plans out. Even He has made mistakes, and you and I are going to remedy that! The Architect of the universe is going to be taught by the carpenters! He has left the world a dirty hole, and you are going to make it a beautiful place!

What is the goal of it all? Can senses ever be the goal? Can enjoyment of pleasure ever be the goal? Can this life ever be the goal of the soul? If it is, better die this moment;

do not want this life! If that is the fate of man, that he is going to be only the perfected machine, it would just mean that we go back to being trees and stones and things like that. Did you ever hear a cow tell a lie or see a tree steal? They are perfect machines. They do not make mistakes. They live in a world where everything is finished.

*

What is the ideal of religion, then, if this cannot be practical [religion]? And it certainly cannot be. What are we here for? We are here for freedom, for knowledge. We want to know in order to make ourselves free. That is our life: one universal cry for freedom.

What is the reason the plant grows from the seed, overturning the ground and raising itself up to the skies? What is the offering for the earth from the sun? What is your life? The same struggle for freedom. Nature is trying all around to suppress us, and the soul wants to express itself.

The struggle with nature is going on. Many things will be crushed and broken in this struggle for freedom. That is your real misery. Large masses of dust and dirt must be raised on the battlefield. Nature says, "I will conquer." The soul says, "I must be the conqueror."

Nature says, "Wait! I will give you a little enjoyment to keep you quiet." The soul enjoys a little, becomes deluded a moment, but the next moment it [cries for freedom again].

Have you marked the eternal cry going on through the ages in every breast? We are deceived by poverty. We become wealthy and are deceived with wealth. We are ignorant. We read and learn and are deceived with knowledge. No man is ever satisfied.

That is the cause of misery, but it is also the cause of all blessing. That is the sure sign. How can you be satisfied with this world? If tomorrow this world becomes heaven, we will say, "Take this away. Give us something else."

*

The infinite human soul can never be satisfied but by the Infinite itself .Infinite desire can only be satisfied by infinite knowledge — nothing short of that.

Worlds will come and go. What of that? The soul lives and for ever expands. Worlds must come into the soul. Worlds must disappear in the soul like drops in the ocean.

And this world to become the goal of the soul! If we have common sense, we cannot he satisfied, though this has been the theme of the poets in all the ages, always telling us to be satisfied. And nobody has been satisfied yet!

Millions of prophets have told us, "Be satisfied with your lot"; poets sing. We have told ourselves to be quiet and satisfied, yet we are not. It is the design of the Eternal that there is nothing in this world to satisfy my soul, nothing in the heavens above, and nothing beneath.

Before the desire of my soul, the stars and the worlds, upper and lower, the whole universe, is but a hateful disease, nothing but that. That is the meaning. Everything is an evil unless that is the meaning. Every desire is evil unless that is the meaning, unless you understand its true importance, its goal. All nature is crying through all the atoms for one thing — its perfect freedom.

*

What is practical religion, then? To get to that state — freedom, the attainment of freedom. And this world, if it helps us on to that goal, [is] all right; if not — if it begins to bind one more layer on the thousands already there, it becomes an evil.

Possessions, learning, beauty, everything else — as long as they help us to that goal, they are of practical value. When they have ceased helping us on to that goal of freedom, they are a positive danger.

What is practical religion, then? Utilise the things of this world and the next just for one goal — the attainment of freedom. Every enjoyment, every ounce of pleasure is to be bought by the expenditure of the infinite heart and mind combined.

Look at the sum total of good and evil in this world. Has it changed? Ages have passed, and practical religion has worked for ages. The world thought that each time the problem would be solved.

It is always the same problem. At best it changes its form. It trades consumption and nerve disease for twenty thousand shops. It is like old rheumatism: Drive it from one place, it goes to another.

A hundred years ago man walked on foot or bought horses. Now he is happy because he rides the railroad; but he is unhappy because he has to work more and earn more. Every machine that saves labour puts more stress upon labour.

This universe, nature, or whatever you call it, must be limited; it can never be unlimited. The Absolute, to become nature, must be limited by time, space, and causation.

The energy [at our disposal] is limited. You can spend it in one place, losing it in another. The sum total is always the same. Wherever there is a wave in one place, there is a hollow in another. If one nation becomes rich, others become poor. Good balances evil. The person for the moment on top of the wave thinks all is good; the person at the bottom says the world is [all evil].

But the man who stands aside sees the divine play going on. Some weep and others laugh. The latter will weep in their turn and the others laugh. What can we do ? We know we cannot do anything.

*

Which of us do anything because we want to do good? How few! They can be counted on the fingers. The rest of us also do good, but because we are forced to do so. We cannot stop. Onward we go, knocked about from place to place.

What can we do? The world will be the same world, the earth the same. It will be changed from blue to brown and from brown to blue. One language translated into another, one set of evils changed into another set of evils — that is what is going on. Six of one, half a dozen of the other.

The American Indian in the forest cannot attend a lecture on metaphysics as you can, but he can digest his meal. You cut him to pieces, and the next moment he is all right. You and I, if we get scratched, we have to go to the hospital for six months.

*

The lower the organism, the greater is its pleasure in the senses. Think of the lowest animals and the power of touch. Everything is touch. When you come to man, you will see that the lower the civilization of the man, the greater is the power of the senses. The higher the organism, the lesser is the pleasure of the senses.

A dog can eat a meal, but cannot understand the exquisite pleasure of thinking about metaphysics. He is deprived of the wonderful pleasure which you get through the intellect. The pleasures of the senses are great.

Greater than those is the pleasure of the intellect. When you attend the fine fifty-course dinner in Paris, that is pleasure indeed. But in the observatory, looking at the stars, seeing worlds coming and developing — think of that!

It must be greater, for I know you forget all about eating. That pleasure must be greater than what you get from worldly things. You forget all about wives, children, husbands, and everything; you forget all about the sense-plane.

That is intellectual pleasure. It is common sense that it must be greater than sense pleasure. It is always for greater joy that you give up the lesser. This is practical religion — the attainment of freedom, renunciation. Renounce!

*

Renounce the lower so that you may get the higher. What is the foundation of society? Morality, ethics, laws.

Renounce. Renounce all temptation to take your neighbour's property, to put hands upon your neighbour, all the pleasure of tyrannising over the weak, all the pleasure of cheating others by telling lies.

Is not morality the foundation of society? What is marriage but the renunciation of unchastity? The savage does not marry. Man marries because he renounces. So on and on.

Renounce! Renounce! Sacrifice! Give up! Not for zero. Not for nothing. But to get the higher.

But who can do this? You cannot, until you have got the higher. You may talk. You may struggle. You may try to do many things. But renunciation comes by itself when you have got the higher. Then the lesser falls away by itself.

*

This is practical religion. What else? Cleaning streets and building hospitals? Their value consists only in this renunciation. And there is no end to renunciation. The difficulty is they try to put a limit to it — thus far and no farther. But there is no limit to this renunciation.

Where God is, there is no other. Where the world is, there is no God. These two will never unite. [Like] light and darkness. That is what I have understood from Christianity and the life of the Teacher.

Is not that Buddhism? Is not that Hinduism? Is not that Mohammedanism? Is not that the teaching of all the great sages and teachers? What is the world that is to be given up? It is here. I am carrying it all with me. My own body. It is all for this body that I put my hand voluntarily upon my fellow man, just to keep it nice and give it a little pleasure; [all for this body] that I injure others and make mistakes.

*

Great men have died. Weak men have died. Gods have died. Death — death everywhere. This world is a graveyard of the infinite past, yet we cling to this [body]: "I am never going to die".

Knowing for sure [that the body must die] and yet clinging to it. There is meaning in that too [because in a sense we do not die]. The mistake is that we cling to the body when it is the spirit that is really immortal.

You are all materialists, because you believe that you are the body. If a man gives me a hard punch, I would say I am punched. If he strikes me, I would say I am struck.

If I am not the body, why should I say so? It makes no difference if I say I am the spirit. I am the body just now. I have converted myself into matter. That is why I am to renounce the body, to go back to what I really am.

I am the spirit — the soul no instrument can pierce, no sword can cut asunder, no fire can burn, no air can dry. Unborn and uncreated, without beginning and without end, deathless, birthless and omnipresent — that is what I am; and all misery comes just because I think this little lump of clay is myself. I am identifying myself with matter and taking all the consequences.

*

Practical religion is identifying myself with my Self. Stop this wrong identification! How far are you advanced in that? You may have built two thousand hospitals, built fifty thousand roads, and yet what of that, if you, have not realised that you are the spirit? You die a dog's; death, with the same feelings that the dog does. The dog howls and weeps because he knows that he is only matter and he is going to be dissolved.

There is death, you know, inevitable death, in water, in air, in the palace, in the prison - death everywhere. What makes you fearless? When you have realised what you are — that infinite spirit, deathless, birthless.

Him no fire can burn, no instrument kill, no poison hurt. Not theory, mind you. Not reading books. [Not parroting.] My old Master used to say, "It is all very good to teach the parrot to say, 'Lord, Lord, Lord' all the time; but let the cat come and take hold of its neck, it forgets all about it."

[You may] pray all the time, read all the scriptures in the world, and worship all the gods there are, [but] unless you realise the soul there is no freedom. Not talking, theorising, argumentation, but realisation. That I call practical religion.

*

This truth about the soul is first to be heard. If you have heard it, think about it. Once you have done that, meditate upon it. No more vain arguments! Satisfy yourself once that you are the infinite spirit. If that is true, it must be nonsense that you are the body.

You are the Self, and that must be realised. Spirit must see itself as spirit. Now the spirit is seeing itself as body. That must stop. The moment you begin to realise that, you are released.

You see this glass, and you know it is simply an illusion. Some scientists tell you it is light and vibration. Seeing the spirit must be infinitely more real: than that, must be the only true state, the only true sensation, the only true vision.

All these [objects you see], are but dreams. You know that now. Not the old idealists alone, but modern physicists also tell you that light is there. A little more vibration makes all the difference.

*

You must see God. The spirit must be realised, and that is practical religion. It is not what Christ preached that you call practical religion: "Blessed are the poor in spirit for theirs is the Kingdom of Heaven."

Was it a joke? What is the practical religion you are thinking, of? Lord help us!

"Blessed are the pure in heart, for they shall see God." That means street-cleaning, hospital-building, and all that? Good works, when you do them with a pure mind.

Don't give the man twenty dollars and buy all the papers in San Francisco to see your name! Don't you read in your own books how no man will help you? Serve as worship of the Lord Himself in the poor, the miserable, the weak. That done, the result is secondary. That sort of work, done without any thought of gain, benefits the soul. And even of such is the Kingdom of Heaven.

*

The Kingdom of Heaven is within us. He is there. He is the soul of all souls. See Him in your own soul. That is practical religion. That is freedom.

Let us ask each other how much we are advanced in that: how much we are worshippers of the body, or real believers in God, the spirit; how much we believe ourselves to be spirit. That is selfless. That is freedom. That is real worship.

Realise yourself. That is all there is to do. Know yourself as you are — infinite spirit. That is practical religion. Everything else is impractical, for everything else will vanish. That alone will never vanish. It Is eternal.

Hospitals will tumble down. Railroad givers will all die. This earth will be blown to pieces, suns wiped out. The soul endureth for ever.

Which is higher, running after these things which perish or. worshipping that which never changes?

Which is more practical, spending all the energies of life in getting things, and before you have got them death comes and you have to leave them all? — like the great [ruler] who conquered all, [who when] death came, said, "Spread out all the jars of things before me."

He said "Bring me that big diamond." And he placed it on his breast and wept. Thus weeping, he died the same as the dog dies.

Man says, "I live." He knows not that it is [the fear of] death that makes him cling slavishly to life. He says "I enjoy." He never dreams that nature has enslaved him.

*

Nature grinds all of us. Keep count of the ounce of pleasure you get. In the long run, nature did her work through you, and when you die your body will make other plants grow. Yet we think all the time that we are getting pleasure ourselves. Thus the wheel goes round.

To realise the spirit as spirit is practical religion. Everything else is good so far as it leads to this one grand idea. That [realization] is to be attained by renunciation, by meditation — renunciation of all the senses, cutting the knots, the chains that bind us down to matter.

Mind

The Being of perfect nature, universally appearing to us, is God, is Absolute. The undifferentiated is the perfect condition; all others must be lower and not permanent.

What makes the undifferentiated appear differentiated to mind? This is the same kind of question as what is the origin of evil and free will?

The question itself is contradictory and impossible, because the question takes for granted cause and effect. There is no cause and effect in the undifferentiated; the question assumes that the undifferentiated is in the same condition as the differentiated. "Whys" and "wherefores" are in mind only.

The Self is beyond causation, and It alone is free. Its light it is which percolates through every form of mind. With every action I assert I am free, and yet every action proves that I am bound.

The real Self is free, yet when mixed with mind and body, It is not free. The will is the first manifestation of the real Self; the first limitation therefore of this real Self is the will. Will is a compound of Self and mind.

Now, no compound can be permanent, so that when we will to live, we must die. Immortal life is a contradiction in terms, for life, being a compound, cannot be immortal. True Being is undifferentiated and eternal.

*

All that is differentiated is nature. Nature is the quality of the plant, the quality of the animal, and the quality of man. Man's life behaves according to definite methods; so does his mind.

Thoughts do not just happen, there is a certain method in their rise, existence and fall. In other words, just as external phenomena are bound by law, internal phenomena, that is to say, the life and mind of man, are also bound by law.

When we consider law in relation to man's mind and existence, it is at once obvious that there can be no such thing as free will and free existence. We know how animal nature is wholly regulated by law.

The animal does not appear to exercise any free will. The same is true of man; human nature also is bound by law. The law governing functions of the human mind is called the law of Karma.

Nobody has ever seen anything produced out of nothing; if anything arises in the mind, that also must have been produced from something. When we speak of free will, we mean the will is not caused by anything.

But that cannot be true, the will is caused; and since it is caused, it cannot be free — it is bound by law. That I am willing to talk to you and you come to listen to me, that is law.

Everything that I do or think or feel, every part of my conduct or behaviour, my every movement — all is caused and therefore not free. This regulation of our life and mind — that is the law of Karma.

If such a doctrine had been introduced in olden times into a Western community, it would have produced a tremendous commotion. The Western man does not want to think his mind is governed by law. In India it was accepted as soon as it was propounded by the most ancient Indian system of philosophy. There is no such thing as freedom of the mind; it cannot be.

*

The Vedas are full of passages which prove the existence of a Personal God. The Rishis, who through long devotion saw God, had a peep into the unknown and threw their challenge to the world.

It is only presumptuous men, who have not walked in the path described by the Rishis and who have not followed their teachings, that criticise them and oppose them. No man has yet come forward who would dare to say that he has properly followed their directions and has not seen anything and that these men are liars.

There are men who have been under trial at various times and have felt that they have not been forsaken by God. The world is such that if faith in God does not offer us any consolation, it is better to commit suicide.

A pious missionary went out on business. All of a sudden his three sons died of cholera. His wife covered the three dead bodies of her beloved children with a sheet and was awaiting her husband at the gate.

When he returned, she detained him at the gate and put him the question, "My dear husband, some one entrusts something to you and in your absence suddenly takes it back. Will you feel sorry?" He replied, "Certainly I would not."

Then she took him in, removed the sheet and showed the three corpses. He bore this calmly and buried the bodies. Such is the strength of mind of those who hold firm faith in the existence of an all – merciful God who disposes of everything in the universe.

The Absolute can never be thought of. We can have no idea of a thing unless it is finite. God the infinite can only be conceived and worshipped as the finite.

*

The greatest power is lodged in the fine, not in the coarse. We see a man take up a huge weight, we see his muscles swell, and all over his body we see signs of exertion, and we think the muscles are powerful things.

But it is the thin thread-like things, the nerves, which bring power to the muscles; the moment one of these threads is cut off from reaching the muscles, they are not able to work at all. These tiny nerves bring the power from something still finer, and that again in its turn brings it from something finer still — thought, and so on. So, it is the fine that is really the seat of power.

Of course we can see the movements in the gross; but when fine movements take place, we cannot see them. When a gross thing moves, we catch it, and thus we naturally identify movement with things which are gross. But all the power is really in the fine. We do not see any movement in the fine, perhaps, because the movement is so intense that we cannot perceive it.

But if by any science, any investigation, we are helped to get hold of these finer forces which are the cause of the expression, the expression itself will be under control. There is a little bubble coming from the bottom of a lake; we do not see it coming all the time, we see it only when it bursts on the surface; so, we can perceive thoughts only after they develop a great deal, or after they become actions.

We constantly complain that we have no control over our actions, over our thoughts. But how can we have it? If we can get control over the fine movements, if we can get hold of thought at the root, before it has become thought, before it has become action, then it would be possible for us to control the whole.

Now, if there is a method by which we can analyse, investigate, understand, and finally grapple with those finer powers, the finer causes, then alone is it possible to have control over ourselves, and the man who has control over his own mind assuredly will have control over every other mind.

That is why purity and morality have been always the object of religion; a pure, moral man has control of himself. And all minds are the same, different parts of one Mind. He who knows one lump of clay has known all the clay in the universe. He who knows and controls his own mind knows the secret of every mind and has power over every mind

*

All these senses, external and internal, must be under the disciple's control. By hard practice he has to arrive at the stage where he can assert his mind against the senses, against the commands of nature. He should be able to say to his mind, "You are mine; I order you, do not see or hear anything", and the mind will not see or hear anything — no form or sound will react on the mind.

In that state the mind has become free of the domination of the senses, has become separated from them. No longer is it attached to the senses and the body. The external things cannot order the mind now; the mind refuses to attach itself to them. Beautiful fragrance is there.

The disciple says to the mind, "Do not smell", and the mind does not perceive the fragrance. When you have arrived at that point, you are just beginning to be a disciple.

That is why when everybody says, "I know the truth", I say, "If you know the truth, you must have self-control; and if you have control of yourself, show it by controlling these organs."

*

Next, the mind must be made to quiet down. It is rushing about. Just as I sit down to meditate, all the vilest subjects in the world come up. The whole thing is nauseating. Why should the mind think thoughts I do not want it to think? I am as it were a slave to the mind.

No spiritual knowledge is possible so long as the mind is restless and out of control. The disciple has to learn to control the mind. Yes, it is the function of the mind to think.

But it must not think if the disciple does not want it to; it must stop thinking when he commands it to. To qualify as a disciple, this state of the mind is very necessary.

*

Also, the disciple must have great power of endurance. Life seems comfortable; and you find the mind behaves well when everything is going well with you.

But if something goes wrong, your mind loses its balance. That is not good. Bear all evil and misery without one murmur of hurt, without one thought of unhappiness, resistance, remedy, or retaliation. That is true endurance; and that you must acquire.

Good and evil there always are in the world. Many forget there is any evil — at least they try to forget; and when evil comes upon them, they are overwhelmed by it and feel bitter.

There are others who deny that there is any evil at all and consider everything good. That also is a weakness; that also proceeds from a fear of evil. If something is evil-smelling, why sprinkle it with rose water and call it fragrant? Yes, there are good and evil in the world — God has put evil in the world. But you do not have to whitewash Him. Why there is evil is none of your business. Please have faith and keep quiet.

*

Without the "I" there can be no "you" outside. From this some philosophers came to the conclusion that the external world did not exist save in the subject; that the "you" existed only in the "I". Others have argued that the "I" can only be known through the "you" and with equal logic.

These two views are partial truths, each wrong in part and each right in part. Thought is as much material and as much in nature as body is. Both matter and mind exist in a third, a unity which divides itself into the two. This unity is the Atman, the real Self.

*

Give up all desire for enjoyment in earth or heaven. Control the organs of the senses and control the mind. Bear every misery without even knowing that you are miserable. Think of nothing but spiritual freedom. Have faith in Guru, in his teachings, and in the surety that you can get free.

Say "Soham, Soham" whatever comes. Tell yourself this even in eating, walking, suffering; tell the mind this incessantly — that what we see never existed, that there is only "I". Flash — the dream will break! Think day and night, this universe is zero, only God is. Have intense desire to get free.

*

Before we can control the mind we must study it. We have to seize this unstable mind and drag it from its wanderings and fix it on one idea. Over and over again this must be done. By power of will we must get hold of the mind and make it stop and reflect upon the glory of God.

The easiest way to get hold of the mind is to sit quiet and let it drift where it will for a while. Hold fast to the idea, "I am the witness watching my mind drifting. The mind is not I." Then see it think as if it were a thing entirely apart from yourself. Identify yourself with God, never with matter or with the mind.

Picture the mind as a calm lake stretched before you and the thoughts that come and go as bubbles rising and breaking on its surface. Make no effort to control the thoughts, but watch them and follow them in imagination as they float away. This will gradually lessen the circles.

For the mind ranges over wide circles of thought and those circles widen out into ever-increasing circles, as in a pond when we throw a stone into it. We want to reverse the process and starting with a huge circle make it narrower until at last we can fix the mind on one point and make it stay there.

Hold to the idea, "I am not the mind, I see that I am thinking, I am watching my mind act", and each day the identification of yourself with thought and feeling will grow less, until at last you can entirely separate yourself from the mind and actually know it to be apart from yourself.

When this is done, the mind is your servant to control as you will. The first stage of being a Yogi is to go beyond the senses. When the mind is conquered, he has reached the highest stage.

*

"If I know one lump of clay, I know the whole mass of clay." The universe is all built on the same plan. The individual is only a part, like the lump of clay. If we know the human soul—which is one atom—its beginning and general history, we know the whole of nature. Birth, growth, development, decay, death—this is the sequence in all nature and is the same in the plant and the man. The difference is only in time.

The whole cycle may be completed in one case in a day, in the other in three score years and ten; the methods are the same. The only way to reach a sure analysis of the universe is by the analysis of our own minds.

A proper psychology is essential to the understanding of religion. To reach Truth by reason alone is impossible, because imperfect reason cannot study its own fundamental basis.

Therefore the only way to study the mind is to get at facts, and then intellect will arrange them and deduce the principles. The intellect has to build the house; but it cannot do so without bricks and it cannot make bricks. Jnana-Yoga is the surest way of arriving at facts.

*

We make a tremendous distinction between matter and mind; we think that the mind is entirely different from matter. Actually, they are but one nature, half of which is continually acting on the other half.

Matter is pressing upon the mind in the form of various sensations. These sensations are nothing but force. The force from the outside evokes the force within. From the will to respond to or get away from the outer force, the inner force becomes what we call thought.

Both matter and mind are really nothing but forces; and if you analyse them far enough, you will find that at root they are one. The very fact that the external force can somehow evoke the internal force shows that somewhere they join each other — they must be continuous and, therefore, basically the same force.

When you get to the root of things, they become simple and general. Since the same force appears in one form as matter and in another form as mind, there is no reason to think matter and mind are different.

Mind is changed into matter, matter is changed into mind. Thought force becomes nerve force, muscular force; muscular and nerve force become thought force. Nature is all this force, whether expressed as matter or mind.

*

The materialist frightens the idealist by claiming to derive his mind from the elements of the laboratory, while all the time he is struggling to express something higher than all elements and atoms, something of which both the external and the internal phenomena are results, and which he terms matter.

The idealist, on the other hand, wants to derive all the elements and atoms of the materialist from his own thought, even while catching glimpses of something which is the cause of both mind and matter, and which he oft-times calls God. That is to say, one party wants to explain the whole universe by a portion of it which is external, the other by another portion which is internal.

Both of these attempts are impossible. Mind and matter cannot explain each other. The only explanation is to be sought for in something which will embrace both matter and mind.

*

Mind is cognised by the Atman, but it is not self-illuminated. The Atman cannot be the cause of anything. How can it be? How can the Purusha join itself to Prakriti (nature)? It does not; it is only illusively thought to do so….

*

The next point is how to use this Prana. We all use it, but how sadly we waste it! The first doctrine in the preparatory stage is that all knowledge is the outcome of experience. Whatever is beyond the five senses must also be experienced in order to become true to us.

Our mind is acting on three planes: the subconscious, conscious, and superconscious. Of men, the Yogi alone is superconscious. The whole theory of Yoga is to go beyond the mind. These three planes can be understood by considering the vibrations of light or sound. There are certain vibrations of light too slow to become visible; then as they get faster, we see them as light; and then they get too fast for us to see them at all. The same with sound.

How to transcend the senses without disturbing the health is what we want to learn. The Western mind has stumbled into acquiring some of the psychic gifts which in them are abnormal and are frequently the sign of disease. The Hindu has studied and made perfect this subject of science, which all may now study without fear or danger.

Mental healing is a fine proof of the superconscious state; for the thought which heals is a sort of vibration in the Prana, and it does not go as a thought but as something higher for which we have no name.

*

Each thought has three states. First, the rising or beginning, of which we are unconscious; second, when the thought rises to the surface; and third, when it goes from us. Thought is like a bubble rising to the surface. When thought is joined to will, we call it power.

That which strikes the sick person whom you are trying to help is not thought, but power. The self-man running through it all is called in Sanskrit Sutrâtmâ, the "Thread-self".

The last and highest manifestation of Prana is love. The moment you have succeeded in manufacturing love out of Prana, you are free. It is the hardest and the greatest thing to gain.

You must not criticise others; you must criticise yourself. If you see a drunkard, do not criticise him; remember he is you in another shape. He who has not darkness sees no darkness in others. What you have inside you is that you see in others.

This is the surest way of reform. If the would-be reformers who criticise and see evil would themselves stop creating evil, the world would be better. Beat this idea into yourself.

*

The modern idea of nature includes only that part of the universe that is manifested on the physical plane. That which is generally understood to be mind is not considered to be nature.

Philosophers endeavouring to prove the freedom of the will have excluded the mind from nature; for as nature is bound and governed by law, strict unbending law, mind, if considered to be in nature, would be bound by law also. Such a claim would destroy the doctrine of free will; for how can that be free which is bound by law?

Law itself is the operation of cause and effect. Certain things happen according to certain other things which have gone before. Every precedent has its consequent.

Thus it is in nature. If this operation of law obtains in the mind, the mind is bound and is therefore not free.

No, the will is not free. How can it be? But we all know, we all feel, that one are free. Life would have no meaning, it would not be worth living, if we were not free.

The Eastern philosophers accepted this doctrine, or rather propounded it, that the mind and the will are within time, space, and causation, the same as so-called matter; and that they are therefore bound by the law of causation. We think in time; our thoughts are bound by time; all that exists, exists in time and space. All is bound by the law of causation.

That which we call matter and mind are one and the same substance. The only difference is in the degree of vibration. Mind at a very low rate of vibration is what is known as matter. Matter at a high rate of vibration is what is known as mind.

Both are the same substance; and therefore, as matter is bound by time and space and causation, mind which is matter at a high rate of vibration is bound by the same law.... Mind becomes matter, and matter in its turn becomes mind, it is simply a question of vibration.

Nature is homogeneous. Differentiation is in manifestation. The Sanskrit word for nature is Prakriti, and means literally differentiation. All is one substance, but it is manifested variously.

Mind becomes matter, and matter in its turn becomes mind, it is simply a question of vibration.

Take a bar of steel and charge it with a force sufficient to cause it to vibrate, and what would happen? If this were done in a dark room, the first thing you would be aware of would be a sound, a humming sound. Increase the force, and the bar of steel would become luminous; increase it still more, and the steel would disappear altogether. It would become mind.

Take another illustration: If I do not eat for ten days, I cannot think. Only a few stray thoughts are in my mind. I am very weak and perhaps do not know my own name.

Then I eat some bread, and in a little while I begin to think; my power of mind has returned. The bread has become mind. Similarly, the mind lessens its rate of vibration and manifests itself in the body, becomes matter.

As to which is first — matter or mind, let me illustrate: A hen lays an egg; the egg brings out another hen; that hen lays another egg; that egg brings out another hen, and so on in an endless chain.

Now which is first — the egg or the hen? You cannot think of an egg that was not laid by a hen, or a hen that was not hatched out of an egg. It makes no difference which is first. Nearly all our ideas run themselves into the hen and egg business.

The greatest truths have been forgotten because of their very simplicity. Great truths are simple because they are of universal application. Truth itself is always simple. Complexity is due to man's ignorance.

*

The book one must read to learn natural sciences is the book of nature. The book from which to learn religion is your own mind and heart. The sage is often ignorant of physical science, because he reads the wrong book — the book within; and the scientist is too often ignorant of religion, because he too reads the wrong book — the book without.

*

Can you tell me where this "I" exists? How can you speak of anything being killed, which never exists at all? Man only remains hypnotised with the false idea of an ego.

When this ghost is off from us, all dreams vanish, and then it is found that the one Self only exists from the highest Being to a blade of grass. This will have to be known, to be realised. All practice or worship is only for taking off this veil.

When that will go, you will find that the Sun of Absolute Knowledge is shining in Its own lustre. For the Atman only is self-luminous and has to be realised by Itself. How can that, which can be experienced only by itself be known with the help of any other thing?

Hence the Shruti says, " — Well, through what means is that to be known which is the Knower?" Whatever you know, you know through the instrumentality of your mind. But mind is something material. It is active only because there is the pure Self behind it.

So, how can you know that Self through your mind? But this only becomes known, after all, that the mind cannot reach the pure Self, no, nor even the intellect. Our relative knowledge ends just there.

Then, when the mind is free from activity or functioning, it vanishes, and the Self is revealed. This state has been described by the commentator Shankara as supersensuous perception.

*

Between the intellect and the grosser matter outside there is only a difference in degree. The Purusha is the only thing which is immaterial.

The mind is an instrument, as it were, in the hands of the soul, through which the soul catches external objects. The mind is constantly changing and vacillating, and can, when perfected, either attach itself to several organs, to one, or to none.

For instance, if I hear the clock with great attention, I will not, perhaps, see anything although my eyes may be open, showing that the mind was not attached to the seeing organ, while it was to the hearing organ. But the perfected mind can be attached to all the organs simultaneously. It has the reflexive power of looking back into its own depths.

This reflexive power is what the Yogi wants to attain; by concentrating the powers of the mind, and turning them inward, he seeks to know what is happening inside. There is in this no question of mere belief; it is the analysis arrived at by certain philosophers.

*

The mind is omnipresent and can be heard and felt anywhere.

*

The science of Raja-Yoga proposes to give us a means of observing the internal states. The instrument is the mind itself. The power of attention, when properly guided, and directed towards the internal world, will analyse the mind, and illumine facts for us.

The powers of the mind are like rays of light dissipated; when they are concentrated, they illumine. This is our only means of knowledge. Everyone is using it, both in the external and the internal world; but, for the psychologist, the same minute observation has to be directed to the internal world, which the scientific man directs to the external; and this requires a great deal of practice.

From our childhood upwards we have been taught only to pay attention to things external, but never to things internal; hence most of us have nearly lost the faculty of observing the internal mechanism.

To turn the mind as it were, inside, stop it from going outside, and then to concentrate all its powers, and throw them upon the mind itself, in order that it may know its own nature, analyse itself, is very hard work. Yet that is the only way to anything which will be a scientific approach to the subject.

*

The purer the mind, the easier it is to control. Purity of the mind must be insisted upon if you would control it. Do not think covetously about mere mental powers. Let them go. One who seeks the powers of the mind succumbs to them. Almost all who desire powers become ensnared by them.

Perfect morality is the all in all of complete control over mind. The man who is perfectly moral has nothing more to do; he is free. The man who is perfectly moral cannot possibly hurt anything or anybody.

Non-injuring has to be attained by him who would be free. No one is more powerful than he who has attained perfect non-injuring. No one could fight, no one could quarrel, in his presence.

Yes, his very presence, and nothing else, means peace, means love wherever he may be. Nobody could be angry or fight in his presence. Even the animals, ferocious animals, would be peaceful before him.

*

I once knew a Yogi, a very old man, who lived in a hole in the ground all by himself. All he had was a pan or two to cook his meals in. He ate very little, and wore scarcely anything, and spent most of his time meditating.

With him all people were alike. He had attained to non-injuring. What he saw in everything, in every person, in every animal, was the Soul, the Lord of the Universe. With him, every person and every animal was "my Lord". He never addressed any person or animal in any other way.

Well, one day a thief came his way and stole one of his pans. He saw him and ran after him. The chase was a long one. At last the thief from exhaustion had to stop, and the Yogi, running up to him, fell on his knees before him and said, "My Lord, you do me a great honour to come my way. Do me the honour to accept the other pan. It is also yours."

This old man is dead now. He was full of love for everything in the world. He would have died for an ant. Wild animals instinctively knew this old man to be their friend. Snakes and ferocious animals would go into his hole and sleep with him. They all loved him and never fought in his presence.

*

The superconscious is the goal. Then when that state is reached, this very man becomes divine, becomes free. And to the mind thus trained to transcend all, gradually this universe will begin to give up its secrets; the book of nature will be read chapter after chapter, till the goal is attained, and we pass from this valley of life and death to that One, where death and life do not exist, and we know the Real and become the Real.

The first thing necessary is a quiet and peaceable life. If I have to go about the world the whole day to make a living, it is hard for me to attain to anything very high in this life. Perhaps in another life I shall be born under more propitious circumstances.

But if I am earnest enough, these very circumstances will change even in this birth. Was there anything you did not get which you really wanted? It could not be. For it is the want that creates the body. It is the light that has bored the holes, as it were, in your head, called the eyes. If the light had not existed, you would have had no eyes. It is sound that had made the ears.

The object of perception existed first, before you made the organ. In a few hundred thousand years or earlier, we may have other organs to perceive electricity and other things. There is no desire for a peaceful mind. Desire will not come unless there is something outside to fulfil it.

*

This mind is a part of the universal mind. Each mind is connected with every other mind. And each mind, wherever it is located, is in actual communication with the whole world.

*

The mind should always go towards God. No other things have any right to withhold it. It should continuously think of God, though this is a very hard task; yet it can be done by persistent practice. What we are now is the result of our past practice.

Again, practice makes us what we shall be. So practice the other way; one sort of turning round has brought us this way, turn the other way and get out of it as soon as you can.

Thinking of the senses has brought us down here — to cry one moment, to rejoice the next, to be at the mercy of every breeze, slave to everything. This is shameful, and yet we call ourselves spirits. Go the other way, think of God; let the mind not think of any physical or mental enjoyment, but of God alone. When it tries to think of anything else, give it a good blow, so that it may turn round and think of God.

As oil poured from one vessel to another falls in an unbroken line, as chimes coming from a distance fall upon the ear as one continuous sound, so should the mind flow towards God in one continuous stream.

We should not only impose this practice on the mind, but the senses too should be employed. Instead of hearing foolish things, we must hear about God; instead of talking foolish words, we must talk of God. Instead of reading foolish books, we must read good ones which tell of God.

*

You are not bound by law. That is in your nature. The mind is in nature and is bound by law. All nature is bound by law, the law of its own action; and this law can never be broken.

If you could break a law of nature, all nature would come to an end in an instant. There would be no more nature. He who attains freedom breaks the law of nature, and for him nature fades away and has no more power over him. Each one will break the law but once and for ever; and that will end his trouble with nature.

Controlling The Mind

How hard it is to control the mind! Well has it been compared to the maddened monkey. There was a monkey, restless by his own nature, as all monkeys are. As if that were not enough some one made him drink freely of wine, so that he became still more restless.

Then a scorpion stung him. When a man is stung by a scorpion, he jumps about for a whole day; so the poor monkey found his condition worse than ever. To complete his misery a demon entered into him. What language can describe the uncontrollable restlessness of that monkey?

The human mind is like that monkey, incessantly active by its own nature; then it becomes drunk with the wine of desire, thus increasing its turbulence. After desire takes possession comes the sting of the scorpion of jealousy at the success of others, and last of all the demon of pride enters the mind, making it think itself of all importance. How hard to control such a mind!

*

The first lesson, then, is to sit for some time and let the mind run on. The mind is bubbling up all the time. It is like that monkey jumping about. Let the monkey jump as much as he can; you simply wait and watch.

Knowledge is power, says the proverb, and that is true. Until you know what the mind is doing you cannot control it. Give it the rein; many hideous thoughts may come into it; you will be astonished that it was possible for you to think such thoughts.

But you will find that each day the mind's vagaries are becoming less and less violent, that each day it is becoming calmer. In the first few months you will find that the mind will have a great many thoughts, later you will find that they have somewhat decreased, and in a few more months they will be fewer and fewer, until at last the mind will be under perfect control; but we must patiently practice every day.

As soon as the steam is turned on, the engine must run; as soon as things are before us we must perceive; so a man, to prove that he is not a machine, must demonstrate that he is under the control of nothing.

This controlling of the mind, and not allowing it to join itself to the centres, is Pratyahara. How is this practised? It is a tremendous work, not to be done in a day. Only after a patient, continuous struggle for years can we succeed.

*

After you have practised Pratyahara for a time, take the next step, the Dhâranâ, holding the mind to certain points. What is meant by holding the mind to certain points? Forcing the mind to feel certain parts of the body to the exclusion of others.

For instance, try to feel only the hand, to the exclusion of other parts of the body. When the Chitta, or mind-stuff, is confined and limited to a certain place it is Dharana. This Dharana is of various sorts, and along with it, it is better to have a little play of the imagination.

For instance, the mind should be made to think of one point in the heart. That is very difficult; an easier way is to imagine a lotus there. That lotus is full of light, effulgent light. Put the mind there. Or think of the lotus in the brain as full of light, or of the different centres in the Sushumna mentioned before.

*

If the mind is not under control, it is no use living in a cave because the same mind will bring all disturbances there. We will find twenty devils in the cave because all the devils are in the mind. If the mind is under control, we can have the cave anywhere, wherever we are.

It is our own mental attitude which makes the world what it is for us. Our thoughts make things beautiful, our thoughts make things ugly. The whole world is in our own minds.

Learn to see things in the proper light. First, believe in this world — that there is meaning behind everything. Everything in the world is good, is holy and beautiful.

If you see something evil, think that you are not understanding it in the right light. Throw the burden on yourselves! Whenever we are tempted to say that the world is going to the dogs, we ought to analyse ourselves, and we shall find that we have lost the faculty of seeing things as they are.

*

The Atman is not to be gained by the weak." If there is no strength in the body and mind, the Atman cannot be realised.

First you have to build the body by good nutritious food — then only will the mind be strong. The mind is but the subtle part of the body. You must retain great strength in your mind and words.

"I am low, I am low" — repeating these ideas in the mind, man belittles and degrades himself.

*

Despondency is not religion, whatever else it may be. By being pleasant always and smiling, it takes you nearer to God, nearer than any prayer. How can those minds that are gloomy and dull love? If they talk of love, it is false; they want to hurt others.

Think of the fanatics; they make the longest faces, and all their religion is to fight against others in word and act. Think of what they have done in the past, and of what they would do now if they were given a free hand. They would deluge the whole world in blood tomorrow if it would bring them power. By worshipping power and making long faces, they lose every bit of love from their hearts.

So the man who always feels miserable will never come to God. It is not religion, it is diabolism to say, "I am so miserable." Every man has his own burden to bear. If you are miserable, try to be happy, try to conquer it.

God is not to be reached by the weak. Never be weak. You must be strong; you have infinite strength within you. How else will you conquer anything? How else will you come to God?

*

"This Atman is not to be attained by the weak", says the Shruti.

Both physical weakness and mental weakness are meant here. "The strong, the hardy" are the only fit students. What can puny, little, decrepit things do? They will break to pieces whenever the mysterious forces of the body and mind are even slightly awakened by the practice of any of the Yogas.

It is "the young, the healthy, the strong" that can score success. Physical strength, therefore, is absolutely necessary. It is the strong body alone that can bear the shock of reaction resulting from the attempt to control the organs.

He who wants to become a Bhakta must be strong, must be healthy. When the miserably weak attempt any of the Yogas, they are likely to get some incurable malady, or they weaken their minds. Voluntarily weakening the body is really no prescription for spiritual enlightenment.

The mentally weak also cannot succeed in attaining the Atman. The person who aspires to be a Bhakta must be cheerful. In the Western world the idea of a religious man is that he never smiles, that a dark cloud must always hang over his face, which, again, must be long drawn with the jaws almost collapsed.

People with emaciated bodies and long faces are fit subjects for the physician, they are not Yogis. It is the cheerful mind that is persevering. It is the strong mind that hews its way through a thousand difficulties. And this, the hardest task of all, the cutting of our way out of the net of Maya, is the work reserved only for giant wills.

*

Yet at the same time excessive mirth should be avoided (Anuddharsha). A mind in that state never becomes calm; it becomes fickle. Excessive merriment will always be followed by sorrow. Tears and laughter are near kin. People so often run from one extreme to the other. Excessive mirth makes us unfit for serious thought. It also fritters away the energies of the mind in vain.

The stronger the will, the less the yielding to the sway of the emotions. Excessive hilarity is quite as objectionable as too much of sad seriousness, and all religious realisation is possible only when the mind is in a steady, peaceful condition of harmonious equilibrium.

Let the mind be cheerful, but calm. Never let it run into excesses, because every excess will be followed by a reaction.

*

The mind uncontrolled and unguided will drag us down, down, for ever—rend us, kill us; and the mind controlled and guided will save us, free us. So it must be controlled, and psychology teaches us how to do it.

To study and analyse any material science, sufficient data are obtained. These facts are studied and analysed and a knowledge of the science is the result. But in the study and analysis of the mind, there are no data, no facts acquired from without, such as are equally at the command of all.

The mind is analysed by itself. The greatest science, therefore, is the science of the mind, the science of psychology.

*

If you intend to study the mind, you must have systematic training; you must practice to bring the mind under your control, to attain to that consciousness from which you will be able to study the mind and remain unmoved by any of its wild gyrations. Otherwise the facts observed will not be reliable; they will not apply to all people and therefore will not be truly facts or data at all.

Among that class who have gone deeply into the study of the mind, the facts observed have been the same, no matter in what part of the world such persons may be or what religious belief they may have. The results obtained by all who go deep enough into the mind are the same.

The mind operates by perception and impulsion. For instance, the rays of the light enter by eyes, are carried by the nerves to the brain, and still I do not see the light. The brain then conveys the impulse to the mind, but yet I do not see the light; the mind then reacts, and the light flashes across the mind. The mind's reaction is impulsion, and as a result the eye perceives the object.

To control the mind, you must go deep down into the subconscious mind, classify and arrange in order all the different impressions, thoughts, etc., stored up there, and control them. This is the first step. By the control of the subconscious mind you get control over the conscious.

Freedom

The idea of happiness without misery, or of life without death, is very good for school-boys and children; but the thinker sees that it is all a contradiction in terms and gives up both. Seek no praise, no reward, for anything you do.

No sooner do we perform a good action than we begin to desire credit for it. No sooner do we give money to some charity than we want to see our names blazoned in the papers. Misery must come as the result of such desires.

The greatest men in the world have passed away unknown. The Buddhas and the Christs that we know are but second-rate heroes in comparison with the greatest men of whom the world knows nothing.

Hundreds of these unknown heroes have lived in every country working silently. Silently they live and silently they pass away; and in time their thoughts find expression in Buddhas or Christs, and it is these latter that become known to us.

The highest men do not seek to get any name or fame from their knowledge. They leave their ideas to the world; they put forth no claims for themselves and establish no schools or systems in their name. Their whole nature shrinks from such a thing.

*

Supposing that freedom is not your nature, by no manner of means can you become free. Supposing you were free and, in some way, you lost that freedom, that shows that you were not free to begin with.

Had you been free, what could have made you lose it? The independent can never be made dependent; if it is really dependent, its independence was a hallucination.

You cannot establish the immortality of the soul, unless you grant that it is by its nature free, or in other words, that it cannot be acted upon by anything outside. For death is an effect produced by some outside cause. I drink poison and I die, thus showing that my body can be acted upon by something outside that is called poison.

But if it be true that the soul is free, it naturally follows that nothing can affect it, and it can never die. Freedom, immortality, blessedness, all depend upon the soul being beyond the law of causation, beyond this Maya.

Of these two which will you take? Either make the first a delusion, or make the second a delusion. Certainly I will make the second a delusion. It is more consonant with all my feelings and aspirations. I am perfectly aware that I am free by nature, and I will not admit that this bondage is true and my freedom a delusion.

*

If you dare declare that you are free, free you are this moment. If you say you are bound, bound you will remain. This is what Advaita boldly declares. I have told you the ideas of the dualists. You can take whichever you like.

*

Slavery is slavery. The chain of gold is quite as bad as the chain of iron. Is there a way out?

It is only the question of memory [of your true nature], not salvation by work. Do you get salvation? You are [already] free.

Go on saying, "I am free". Never mind if the next moment delusion comes and says, "I am bound." Dehypnotise the whole thing.

[This truth] is first to be heard. Hear it first. Think on it day and night. Fill the mind [with it] day and night: "I am It. I am the Lord of the universe. Never was there any delusion. "

Meditate upon it with all the strength of the mind till you actually see these walls, houses, everything, melt away — [until] body, everything, vanishes. "I will stand alone. I am the One."

Struggle on! "Who cares! We want to be free; [we] do not want any powers. Worlds we renounce; heavens we renounce; hells we renounce. What do I care about all these powers, and this and that! What do I care if the mind is controlled or uncontrolled! Let it run on. What of that! I am not the mind, Let it go on!"

*

When we free ourselves from name and form, especially from a body — when we need no body, good or bad — then only do we escape from bondage. Eternal progression is eternal bondage; annihilation of form is to be preferred. We must get free from any body, even a "god-body". God is the only real existence, there cannot be two. There is but One Soul, and I am That.

*

All nature is crying through all the atoms for one thing — its perfect freedom. However mistaken we may be as to the method, all our struggle is really for freedom We seek neither misery nor happiness, but freedom, freedom alone. This one aim is the secret of the insatiable thirst of man.

*

Freedom in all matters, i.e. advance towards Mukti is the worthiest gain of man. To advance oneself towards freedom — physical, mental, and spiritual — and help others to do so, is the supreme prize of man.

Those social rules which stand in the way of the unfoldment of this freedom are injurious, and steps should be taken to destroy them speedily. Those institutions should be encouraged by which men advance in the path of freedom.

*

Freedom is inseparably connected with immortality. To be free one must be above the laws of nature. Law exists so long as we are ignorant. When knowledge comes, then we find that law nothing but freedom in ourselves.

The will can never be free, because it is the slave of cause and effect. But the "I" behind the will is free; and this is the Self. "I am free" — that is the basis on which to build and live. And freedom means immortality.

*

Work is inevitable, it must be so; but we should work to the highest purpose. Karma-Yoga makes us admit that this world is a world of five minutes, that it is a something we have to pass through; and that freedom is not here, but is only to be found beyond.

To find the way out of the bondages of the world we have to go through it slowly and surely. There may be those exceptional persons about whom I just spoke, those who can stand aside and give up the world, as a snake casts off its skin and stands aside and looks at it. There are no doubt these exceptional beings; but the rest of mankind have to go slowly through the world of work. Karma-Yoga shows the process, the secret, and the method of doing it to the best advantage.

What does it say? "Work incessantly, but give up all attachment to work."

*

Freedom is of the nature of the soul, it is its birthright: that real freedom of the soul shines through veils of matter in the form of the apparent freedom of man.

Every moment of your life you feel that you are free. We cannot live, talk, or breathe for a moment without feeling that we are free; but, at the same time, a little thought shows us that we are like machines and not free.

What is true then? Is this idea of freedom a delusion? One party holds that the idea of freedom is a delusion; another says that the idea of bondage is a delusion.

How does this happen? Man is really free, the real man cannot but be free. It is when he comes into the world of Maya, into name and form, that he becomes bound.

Free will is a misnomer. Will can never be free. How can it be? It is only when the real man has become bound that his will comes into existence, and not before. The will of man is bound, but that which is the foundation of that will is eternally free.

So, even in the state of bondage which we call human life or god-life, on earth or in heaven, there yet remains to us that recollection of the freedom which is ours by divine right. And consciously or unconsciously we are all struggling towards it. When a man has attained his own freedom, how can he be bound by any law? No law in this universe can bind him, for this universe itself is his.

*

I was once travelling in the desert in India. I travelled for over a month and always found the most beautiful landscapes before me, beautiful lakes and all that.

One day I was very thirsty and I wanted to have a drink at one of these lakes; but when I approached that lake it vanished. Immediately with a blow came into my brain the idea that this was a mirage about which I had read all my life; and then I remembered and smiled at my folly, that for the last month all the beautiful landscapes and lakes I had been seeing were this mirage, but I could not distinguish them then.

The next morning I again began my march; there was the lake and the landscape, but with it immediately came the idea, "This is a mirage."

Once known it had lost its power of illusion. So this illusion of the universe will break one day. The whole of this will vanish, melt away. This is realisation.

*

According to the Advaita philosophy, then, this differentiation of matter, these phenomena, are, as it were, for a time, hiding the real nature of man; but the latter really has not been changed at all. In the lowest worm, as well as in the highest human being, the same divine nature is present.

The worm form is the lower form in which the divinity has been more overshadowed by Maya; that is the highest form in which it has been least overshadowed. Behind everything the same divinity is existing, and out of this comes the basis of morality.

Do not injure another. Love everyone as your own self, because the whole universe is one. In injuring another, I am injuring myself; in loving another, I am loving myself.

From this also springs that principle of Advaita morality which has been summed up in one word — self-abnegation. The Advaitist says, this little personalised self is the cause of all my misery.

This individualised self, which makes me different from all other beings, brings hatred and jealousy and misery, struggle and all other evils. o this is to be given up. We must always hold ourselves ready, even to give up our lives for the lowest beings.

When a man has become ready even to give up his life for a little insect, he has reached the perfection which the Advaitist wants to attain; and at that moment when he has become thus ready, the veil of ignorance falls away from him, and he will feel his own nature.

Even in this life, he will feel that he is one with the universe. For a time, as it were, the whole of this phenomenal world will disappear for him, and he will realise what he is. But so long as the Karma of this body remains, he will have to live.

This state, when the veil has vanished and yet the body remains for some time, is what the Vedantists call the Jivanmukti, the living freedom.

*

The mind is not the body, though it is matter in a finer form. It is not eternally bound by the body. This is proved as we get occasionally loosened from it. We can learn to do this at will by controlling the senses.

When we can do that fully, we shall control the universe, because our world is only what the senses bring us. Freedom is the test of the higher being. Spiritual life begins when you have loosened yourself from the control of the senses. He whose senses rule him is worldly — is a slave.

If we could entirely stop our mind-stuff from breaking into waves, it would put an end to our bodies. For millions of years we have worked so hard to manufacture these bodies that in the struggle we have forgotten our real purpose in getting them, which was to become perfect.

We have grown to think that body-making is the end of our efforts. This is Mâyâ. We must break this delusion and return to our original aim and realise we are not the body, it is our servant.

*

Freedom of the will — it is as you feel you are free to act. But this freedom is a species of necessity. There is one infinite link before, after, and between the thought and the action, but the latter takes the name of freedom — like a bird flitting through a bright room. We feel the freedom and feel it has no other cause.

We cannot go beyond consciousness, therefore we feel we are free. We can trace it no further than consciousness. God alone feels the real freedom. Mahapurushas (saints) feel themselves identified with God; hence they also feel the real freedom.

You may stop the water flowing out of the fountain by closing that part of the stream and gathering it all in the fountain; you have no liberty beyond it. But the source remains unchanged.

Everything is predestination — and a part of that predestination is that you shall have such feeling — the feeling of freedom. I am shaping my own action. Responsibility is the feeling of reaction. There is no absolute power. Power here is the conscious feeling of exercising any faculty which is created by necessity.

Man has the feeling "I act"; what he means by power of freedom is the feeling. The power is attended with responsibility. Whatever may be done through us by predestination, we feel the reaction. A ball thrown by one, itself feels the reaction.

But this innate necessity which comes to us as our freedom does not affect also the conscious relations we form with our surroundings. The relativity is not changed. Either everybody is free or everybody is under necessity. That would not matter. The relations would be the same. Vice and virtue would be the same.

If a thief pleads that he was under the necessity of stealing, the magistrate would say that he was under the necessity to punish. We are seated in a room, and the whole room is moving — the relation between us is unchanged.

To get out of this infinite chain of causation is Mukti (freedom). Muktas (free souls) are not actuated by necessity, they are like god. They begin the chain of cause and effect. God is the only free being — the first source of their will — and is always experienced by them as such.

The feeling of want is the real prayer, not the words. But you must have patience to wait and see if your prayers are answered.

*

We have a place for struggle in the Vedanta, but not for fear. All fears will vanish when you begin to assert your own nature. If you think that you are bound, bound you will remain. If you think you are free, free you will be.

That sort of freedom which we can feel when we are yet in the phenomenal is a glimpse of the real but not yet the real.

I disagree with the idea that freedom is obedience to the laws of nature. I do not understand what it means. According to the history of human progress, it is disobedience to nature that has constituted that progress.

It may be said that the conquest of lower laws was through the higher. But even there, the conquering mind was only trying to be free; and as soon as it found that the struggle was also through law, it wanted to conquer that also. So the ideal was freedom in every case.

The trees never disobey law. I never saw a cow steal. An oyster never told a lie. Yet they are not greater than man. This life is a tremendous assertion of freedom; and this obedience to law, carried far enough, would make us simply matter — either in society, or in politics, or in religion.

Too many laws are a sure sign of death. Wherever in any society there are too many laws, it is a sure sign that that society will soon die. If you study the characteristics of India, you will find that no nation possesses so many laws as the Hindus, and national death is the result.

But the Hindus had one peculiar idea — they never made any doctrines or dogmas in religion; and the latter has had the greatest growth. Eternal law cannot be freedom, because to say that the eternal is inside law is to limit it.

*

The atmosphere of a room may be hypnotised so that everybody who enters it will see all sorts of things — men and objects flying through the air.

Everybody is hypnotised already. The work of attaining freedom, of realising one's real nature, consists in de-hypnotisation.

One thing to be remembered is that we are not gaining powers at all. We have them already. The whole process of growth is de-hypnotisation.

*

Only freedom can produce true morality. If there were only an endless chain of cause and effect, Nirvâna could not be. It is extinction of the seeming self, bound by this chain. That is what constitutes freedom, to get beyond causality.

*

Everything that we perceive around us is struggling towards freedom, from the atom to the man, from the insentient, lifeless particle of matter to the highest existence on earth, the human soul. The whole universe is in fact the result of this struggle for freedom.

In all combinations every particle is trying to go on its own way, to fly from the other particles; but the others are holding it in check. Our earth is trying to fly away from the sun, and the moon from the earth.

Everything has a tendency to infinite dispersion. All that we see in the universe has for its basis this one struggle towards freedom; it is under the impulse of this tendency that the saint prays and the robber robs. When the line of action taken is not a proper one, we call it evil; and when the manifestation of it is proper and high, we call it good.

But the impulse is the same, the struggle towards freedom. The saint is oppressed with the knowledge of his condition of bondage, and he wants to get rid of it; so he worships God. The thief is oppressed with the idea that he does not possess certain things, and he tries to get rid of that want, to obtain freedom from it; so he steals.

Freedom is the one goal of all nature, sentient or insentient; and consciously or unconsciously, everything is struggling towards that goal. The freedom which the saint seeks is very different from that which the robber seeks; the freedom loved by the saint leads him to the enjoyment of infinite, unspeakable bliss, while that on which the robber has set his heart only forges other bonds for his soul.

*

Bondage and liberty, light and shadow, good and evil must be there, but the very fact of the bondage shows also this freedom hidden there. If one is a fact, the other is equally a fact. There must be this idea of freedom.

While now we cannot see that this idea of bondage, in uncultivated man, is his struggle for freedom, yet the idea of freedom is there. The bondage of sin and impurity in the uncultivated savage is to his consciousness very small, for his nature is only a little higher than the animal's. What he struggles against is the bondage of physical nature, the lack of physical gratification, but out of this lower consciousness grows and broadens the higher conception of a mental or moral bondage and a longing for spiritual freedom.

Here we see the divine dimly shining through the veil of ignorance. The veil is very dense at first and the light may be almost obscured, but it is there, ever pure and undimmed — the radiant fire of freedom and perfection. Man personifies this as the Ruler of the Universe, the One Free Being. He does not yet know that the universe is all one, that the difference is only in degree, in the concept.

Freedom is the Goal

Our main problem is to be free. It is evident then that until we realise ourselves as the Absolute, we cannot attain to deliverance.

Yet there are various ways of attaining to this realisation. These methods have the generic name of Yoga (to join, to join ourselves to our reality). These Yogas, though divided into various groups, can principally be classed into four; and as each is only a method leading indirectly to the realisation of the Absolute, they are suited to different temperaments.

Now it must be remembered that it is not that the assumed man becomes the real man or Absolute. There is no becoming with the Absolute. It is ever free, ever perfect; but the ignorance that has covered Its nature for a time is to be removed.

Therefore the whole scope of all systems of Yoga (and each religion represents one) is to clear up this ignorance and allow the Âtman to restore its own nature. The chief helps in this liberation are Abhyâsa and Vairâgya. Vairagya is non-attachment to life, because it is the will to enjoy that brings all this bondage in its train; and Abhyasa is constant practice of any one of the Yogas.

*

Love is God, freedom is God; and everything that is bondage is not God.

Man has freedom already, but he will have to discover it. He has it, but every moment forgets it. That discovering, consciously or unconsciously, is the whole life of every one.

But the difference between the sage and the ignorant man is that one does it consciously and the other unconsciously. Every one is struggling for freedom — from the atom to the star. The ignorant man is satisfied if he can get freedom within a certain limit — if he can get rid of the bondage of hunger or of being thirsty.

But that sage feels that there is a stronger bondage which has to be thrown off. He would not consider the freedom of the Red Indian as freedom at all.

*

According to our philosophers, freedom is the goal. Knowledge cannot be the goal, because knowledge is a compound. It is a compound of power and freedom, and it is freedom alone that is desirable. That is what men struggle after.

Simply the possession of power would not be knowledge. For instance, a scientist can send an electric shock to a distance of some miles; but nature can send it to an unlimited distance.

Why do we not build statues to nature then? It is not law that we want but ability to break law. We want to be outlaws. If you are bound by laws, you will be a lump of clay. Whether you are beyond law or not is not the question; but the thought that we are beyond law — upon that is based the whole history of humanity.

For instance, a man lives in a forest, and never has had any education or knowledge. He sees a stone falling down — a natural phenomenon happening — and he thinks it is freedom. He thinks it has a soul, and the central idea in that is freedom.

But as soon as he knows that it must fall, he calls it nature — dead, mechanical action. I may or may not go into the street. In that is my glory as a man. If I am sure that I must go there, I give myself up and become a machine. Nature with its infinite power is only a machine; freedom alone constitutes sentient life.

The Vedanta says that the idea of the man in the forest is the right one; his glimpse is right, but the explanation is wrong. He holds to this nature as freedom and not as governed by law.

Uniformity of action is what we call law. This uniformity of my actions, I find, is broken into very short periods, and so I do not call my actions under law. I work through freedom. I walk for five minutes; but before those five minutes of walking, which are uniform, there was the action of the will, which gave the impulse to walk.

Therefore man says he is free, because all his actions can be cut up into small periods; and although there is sameness in the small periods, beyond the period there is not the same sameness. In this perception of non-uniformity is the idea of freedom.

In nature we see only very large periods of uniformity; but the beginning and end must be free impulses. The impulse of freedom was given just at the beginning, and that has rolled on; but this, compared with our periods, is much longer.

We find by analysis on philosophic grounds that we are not free. But there will remain this factor, this consciousness that I am free. What we have to explain is, how that comes.

We will find that we have these two impulsions in us. Our reason tells us that all our actions are caused, and at the same time, with every impulse we are asserting our freedom. The solution of the Vedanta is that there is freedom inside — that the soul is really free — but that that soul's actions are percolating through body and mind, which are not free.

As soon as we react, we become slaves. A man blames me, and I immediately react in the form of anger. A little vibration which he created made me a slave. So we have to demonstrate our freedom.

*

All things in nature work according to law. Nothing is excepted. The mind as well as everything in external nature is governed and controlled by law.

Internal and external nature, mind and matter, are in time and space, and are bound by the law of causation.

The freedom of the mind is a delusion. How can the mind be free when it is controlled and bound by law?

The law of Karma is the law of causation.

We must become free. We are free; the work is to know it. We must give up all slavery, all bondage of whatever kind. We must not only give up our bondage to earth and everything and everybody on earth, but also to all ideas of heaven and happiness.

We are bound to earth by desire and also to God, heaven, and the angels. A slave is a slave whether to man, to God, or to angels.

The idea of heaven must pass away. The idea of heaven after death where the good live a life of eternal happiness is a vain dream, without a particle of meaning or sense in it.

Wherever there is happiness there must follow unhappiness sometime. Wherever there is pleasure there must be pain. This is absolutely certain, every action has its reaction somehow.

The idea of freedom is the only true idea of salvation — freedom from everything, the senses, whether of pleasure or pain, from good as well as evil.

More than this even, we must be free from death and to be free from death, we must be free from life. Life is but a dream of death. Where there is life, there will be death; so get away from life if you would be rid of death.

We are ever free if we would only believe it, only have faith enough. You are the soul, free and eternal, ever free ever blessed. Have faith enough and you will be free in a minute.

Everything in time, space, and causation is bound. The soul is beyond all time, all space, all causation. That which is bound is nature, not the soul.

Therefore proclaim your freedom and be what you are — ever free, ever blessed.

Time, space, and causation we call Maya.

*

The goal of all nature is freedom, and freedom is to be attained only by perfect unselfishness; every thought, word, or deed that is unselfish takes us towards the goal, and, as such, is called moral. That definition, you will find, holds good in every religion and every system of ethics.

The End of All Bondage

There was never a human race which did not have a religion and worship some sort of God or gods. Whether the God or gods existed or not is no question; but what is the analysis of this psychological phenomenon?

Why is all the world trying to find, or seeking for, a God? Why?

Because in spite of all this bondage, in spite of nature and this tremendous energy of law grinding us down, never allowing us to turn to any side — wherever we go, whatever we want to do, we are thwarted by this law, which is everywhere — in spite of all this, the human soul never forgets its freedom and is ever seeking it. The search for freedom is the search of all religions; whether they know it or not, whether they can formulate it well or ill, the idea is there.

Even the lowest man, the most ignorant, seeks for something which has power over nature's laws. He wants to see a demon, a ghost, a god — somebody who can subdue nature, for whom nature is not almighty, for whom there is no law.

"Oh, for somebody who can break the law!" That is the cry coming from the human heart. We are always seeking for someone who breaks the law.

The rushing engine speeds along the railway track; the little worm crawls out of its way. We at once say, "The engine is dead matter, a machine; and the worm is alive," because the worm attempted to break the law. The engine, with all its power and might, can never break the law. It is made to go in any direction man wants, and it cannot do otherwise; but the worm, small and little though it was, attempted to break the law and avoid the danger. It tried to assert itself against law, assert its freedom; and there was the sign of the future God in it.

Everywhere we see this assertion of freedom, this freedom of the soul. It is reflected in every religion in the shape of God or gods; but it is all external yet — for those who only see the gods outside.

Man decided that he was nothing. He was afraid that he could never be free; so he went to seek for someone outside of nature who was free. Then he thought that there were many and many such free beings, and gradually he merged them all into one God of gods and Lord of lords.

Even that did not satisfy him. He came a little closer to truth, a little nearer; and then gradually found that whatever he was, he was in some way connected with the God of gods and Lord of lords; that he, though he thought himself bound and low and weak, was somehow connected with that God of gods.

Then visions came to him; thought arose and knowledge advanced. And he began to come nearer and nearer to that God, and at last found out that God and all the gods, this whole psychological phenomenon connected with the search for an all-powerful free soul, was but a reflection of his own idea of himself.

And then at last he discovered that it was not only true that "God made man after His own image", but that it was also true that man made God after his own image. That brought out the idea of divine freedom. The Divine Being was always within, the nearest of the near.

Him we had ever been seeking outside, and at last found that He is in the heart of our hearts. You may know the story of the man who mistook his own heartbeat for somebody knocking at the door, and went to the door and opened it, but found nobody there, so he went back.

Again he seemed to hear a knocking at the door, but nobody was there. Then he understood that it was his own heartbeat, and he had misinterpreted it as a knocking at the door.

Similarly, man after his search finds out that this infinite freedom that he was placing in imagination all the time in the nature outside is the internal subject, the eternal Soul of souls; this Reality, he himself.

Thus at last he comes to recognise this marvellous duality of existence: the subject, infinite and finite in one — the Infinite Being is also the same finite soul. The Infinite is caught, as it were, in the meshes of the intellect and apparently manifests as finite beings, but the reality remains unchanged.

This is, therefore, true knowledge: that the Soul of our souls, the Reality that is within us, is That which is unchangeable, eternal, ever-blessed, ever-free. This is the only solid ground for us to stand upon.

This, then, is the end of all death, the advent of all immortality, the end of all misery. And he who sees that One among the many, that One unchangeable in the universe of change, he who sees Him as the Soul of his soul, unto him belongs eternal peace — unto none else.

Faith in God

A man must not only have faith but intellectual faith too. To make a man take up everything and believe it, would be to make him a lunatic.

I once had a book sent me, which said I must believe everything told in it. It said there was no soul, but that there were gods and goddesses in heaven, and a thread of light going from each of our heads to heaven!

How did the writer know all these things? She had been inspired, and wanted me to believe it too; and because I refused, she said, "You must be a very bad man; there is no hope for you!" This is fanaticism.

*

Never say man is weak. Wisdom-Yoga is no better than the others. Love is the ideal and requires no object. Love is God. So even through devotion we reach the subjective God. I am He!

How can one work, unless one loves city, country, animals, the universe? Reason leads to the finding of unity in variety. Let the atheist and the agnostic work for the social good. So God comes.

But this you must guard against: Do not disturb the faith of any. For you must know that religion is not in doctrines. Religion lies in being and becoming, in realisation.

All men are born idolaters. The lowest man is an animal. The highest man is perfect. And between these two, all have to think in sound and colour, in doctrine and ritual.

The test of having ceased to be an idolater is: "When you say 'I', does the body come into your thought or not? If it does, then you are still a worshipper of idols."

Religion is not intellectual jargon at all, but realisation. If you think about God, you are only a fool. The ignorant man, by prayer and devotion, can reach beyond the philosopher.

To know God, no philosophy is necessary. Our duty is not to disturb the faith of others. Religion is experience.

Above all and in all, be sincere; identification brings misery, because it brings desire. Thus the poor man sees gold, and identifies himself with the need of gold. Be the witness. Learn never to react .

*

There is no external test for inspiration, we know it ourselves; our guardian against mistake is negative — the voice of reason. All religion is going beyond reason, but reason is the only guide to get there.

Instinct is like ice, reason is the water, and inspiration is the subtlest form or vapour; one follows the other. Everywhere is this eternal sequence — unconsciousness, consciousness, intelligence — matter, body, mind — and to us it seems as if the chain began with the particular link we first lay hold of.

Arguments on both sides are of equal weight, and both are true. We must reach beyond both, to where there is neither the one nor the other. These successions are all Maya.

Religion is above reason, supernatural. Faith is not belief, it is the grasp on the Ultimate, an illumination. First hear, then reason and find out all that reason can give about the Atman; let the flood of reason flow over It, then take what remains.

If nothing remains, thank God you have escaped a superstition. When you have determined that nothing can take away the Atman, that It stands every test, hold fast to this and teach it to all. Truth cannot be partial; it is for the good of all.

Finally, in perfect rest and peace meditate upon It, concentrate your mind upon It, make yourself one with It. Then no speech is needed; silence will carry the truth.

Do not spend your energy in talking, but meditate in silence; and do not let the rush of the outside world disturb you. When your mind is in the highest state, you are unconscious of it. Accumulate power in silence and become a dynamo of spirituality.

What can a beggar give? Only a king can give, and he only when he wants nothing himself.

*

Work hard, be steady, and have faith in the Lord. Set to work.

You know the disease, you know the remedy, only have faith. Do not look up to the so-called rich and great; do not care for the heartless intellectual writers, and their cold-blooded newspaper articles.

Oneness With God

Through freedom the sciences were built; and in them we have two sets of opinions, the one the materialistic and denouncing, and the other the positive and constructive. It is a most curious fact that in every society you find them.

Supposing there is an evil in society, you will find immediately one group rise up and denounce it in vindictive fashion, which sometimes degenerates into fanaticism. There are fanatics in every society, and women frequently join in these outcries, because of their impulsive nature.

Every fanatic who gets up and denounces something can secure a following. It is very easy to break down; a maniac can break anything he likes, but it would be hard for him to build up anything. These fanatics may do some good, according to their light, but much more harm. Because social institutions are not made in a day, and to change them means removing the cause.

Suppose there is an evil; denouncing it will not remove it, but you must go to work at the root. First find out the cause, then remove it, and the effect will be removed also. Mere outcry not produce any effect, unless indeed it produces misfortune.

*

There are others who had sympathy in their hearts and who understood the idea that we must go deep into the cause, these were the great saints. One fact you must remember, that all the great teachers of the world have declared that they came not to destroy but to fulfil.

Many times, his has not been understood, and their forbearance has been thought to be an unworthy compromise with existing popular opinions. Even now, you occasionally hear that these prophets and great teachers were rather cowardly, and dared not say and do what they thought was right; but that was not so.

Fanatics little understand the infinite power of love in the hearts of these great sages who looked upon the inhabitants of this world as their children. They were the real fathers, the real gods, filled with infinite sympathy and patience for everyone; they were ready to bear and forbear. They knew how human society should grow, and patiently slowly, surely, went on applying their remedies, not by denouncing and frightening people, but by gently and kindly leading them upwards step by step.

Such were the writers of the Upanishads. They knew full well how the old ideas of God were not reconcilable with the advanced ethical ideas of the time; they knew full well that what the atheists were preaching contained a good deal of truth, nay, great nuggets of truth; but at the same time, they understood that those who wished to sever the thread that bound the beads, who wanted to build a new society in the air, would entirely fail.

We never build anew, we simply change places; we cannot have anything new, we only change the position of things. The seed grows into the tree, patiently and gently;

we must direct our energies towards the truth and fulfil the truth that exists, not try to make new truths.

Thus, instead of denouncing these old ideas of God as unfit for modern times, the ancient sages began to seek out the reality that was in them. The result was the Vedanta philosophy, and out of the old deities, out of the monotheistic God, the Ruler of the universe, they found yet higher and higher ideas in what is called the Impersonal Absolute; they found oneness throughout the universe.

He who sees in this world of manifoldness that One running through all, in this world of death he who finds that One Infinite Life, and in this world of insentience and ignorance he who finds that One Light and Knowledge, unto him belongs eternal peace. Unto none else, unto none else.

*

The people of old knew that fire lived in the flint and in dry wood, but friction was necessary to call it out. So this fire of freedom and purity is the nature of every soul, and not a quality, because qualities can be acquired and therefore can be lost.

The soul is one with Freedom, and the soul is one with Existence, and the soul is one with Knowledge. The Sat-Chit-Ânanda — Existence-Knowledge-Bliss Absolute — is the nature, the birthright of the Soul, and all the manifestations that we see are Its expressions, dimly or brightly manifesting Itself. Even death is but a manifestation of that Real Existence.

Birth and death, life and decay, degeneration and regeneration — are all manifestations of that Oneness. So, knowledge, however it manifests itself, either as ignorance or as learning, is but the manifestation of that same Chit, the essence of knowledge; the difference is only in degree, and not in kind.

The difference in knowledge between the lowest worm that crawls under our feet and the highest genius that the world may produce is only one of degree, and not of kind. The Vedantin thinker boldly says that the enjoyments in this life, even the most degraded joys, are but manifestations of that One Divine Bliss, the Essence of the Soul.

*

We believe in one God, the Father of us all, who is omnipresent and omnipotent, and who guides and preserves His children with infinite love. We believe in a Personal God as the Christians do, but we go further: we below that we are He!

That His personality is manifested in us, that God is in us, and that we are in God. We believe there is a germ of truth in all religions, and the Hindu bows down to them all; for in this world, truth is to be found not in subtraction but in addition.

We would offer God a bouquet of the most beautiful flowers of all the diverse faiths. We must love God for love's sake, not for the hope of reward. We must do our duty for duty's sake not for the hope of reward. We must worship the beautiful for beauty's sake, not for the hope of reward.

Thus in the purity of our hearts shall we see God. Sacrifices genuflexions, mumblings, and mutterings are not religion. They are only good if they stimulate us to the brave performance of beautiful and heroic deeds and lift our thoughts to the apprehension of the divine perfection

What good is it, if we acknowledge in our prayers that God is the Father of us all, and in our daily lives do not treat every man as our brother? Books are only made so that they may point the way to a higher life; but no good results unless the path is trodden with unflinching steps!

Every human personality may be compared to a glass globe. There is the same pure white light — an emission of the divine Being — in the centre of each, but the glass being of different colours and thickness, the rays assume diverse aspects in the transmission.

The equality and beauty of each central flame is the same, and the apparent inequality is only in the imperfection of the temporal instrument of its expression. As we rise higher and higher in the scale of being, the medium becomes more and more translucent.

What we want is not so much spirituality as a little of the bringing down of the Advaita into the material world. First bread and then religion. We stuff them too much with religion, when the poor fellows have been starving. No dogmas will satisfy the cravings of hunger.

There are two curses here: first our weakness, secondly, our hatred, our dried-up hearts.

You may talk doctrines by the millions, you may have sects by the hundreds of millions; ay, but it is nothing until you have the heart to feel. Feel for them as your Veda teaches you, till you find they are parts of your own bodies, till you realise that you and they, the poor and the rich, the saint and the sinner, are all parts of One Infinite Whole, which you call Brahman.

"He goes from death to death who sees the many here." See that One and be free.

How are we to see it? This mind, so deluded, so weak, so easily led, even this mind can be strong and may catch a glimpse of that knowledge, that Oneness, which saves us from dying again and again.

As rain falling upon a mountain flow in various streams down the sides of the mountain, so all the energies which you see here are from that one Unit. It has become manifold falling upon Maya. Do not run after the manifold; go towards the One.

"He is in all that moves; He is in all that is pure; He fills the universe; He is in the sacrifice; He is the guest in the house; He is in man, in water, in animals, in truth; He is the Great One. As fire coming into this world is manifesting itself in various forms, even so, that one Soul of the universe is manifesting Himself in all these various forms. As air coming into this universe manifests itself in various forms, even so, the One Soul of all souls, of all beings, is manifesting Himself in all forms."

This is true for you when you have understood this Unity, and not before Then is all optimism, because He is seen everywhere.

The question is that if all this be true that that Pure One — the Self, the Infinite — has entered all this, how is it that He suffers, how is it that He becomes miserable, impure?

He does not, says the Upanishad. "As the sun is the cause of the eyesight of every being, yet is not made defective by the defect in any eye, even so the Self of all is not affected by the miseries of the body, or by any misery that is around you."

I may have some disease and see everything yellow, but the sun is not affected by it.

"He is the One, the Creator of all, the Ruler of all, the Internal Soul of every being — He who makes His Oneness manifold. Thus sages who realise Him as the Soul of their souls, unto them belongs eternal peace; unto none else, unto none else. He who in this world of evanescence finds Him who never changes, he who in this universe of death finds that One Life, he who in this manifold finds that Oneness, and all those who realise Him as the Soul of their souls, to them belongs eternal peace; unto none else, unto none else. Where to find Him in the external world, where to find Him in the suns, and moons, and stars? There the sun cannot illumine, nor the moon, nor the stars, the flash of lightning cannot illumine the place; what to speak of this mortal fire? He shining, everything else shines. It is His light that they have borrowed, and He is shining through them."

Here is another beautiful simile. Those of you who have been in India and have seen how the banyan tree comes from one root and spreads itself far around, will understand this.

He is that banyan tree; He is the root of all and has branched out until He has become this universe, and however far He extends, every one of these trunks and branches is connected.

"He the Omnipresent, the One without a second, the One without a body, pure, the great poet of the universe, whose metre is the suns and stars, is giving to each what he deserves" (Isha Upanishad, 8, adapted).

"He, the One, who vibrates more quickly than mind, who attains to more speed than mind can ever do, whom even the gods reach not, nor thought grasps, He moving, everything moves. In Him all exists. He is moving. He is also immovable. He is near and He is far. He is inside everything. He is outside everything, interpenetrating everything. Whoever sees in every being that same Atman, and whoever sees everything in that Atman, he never goes far from that Atman. When all life and the whole universe are seen in this Atman, then alone man has attained the secret. There is no more delusion for him. Where is any more misery for him who sees this Oneness in the universe?"

The seer is really the Self, the pure one, the ever holy, the infinite, the immortal. This is the Self of man. And what are the instruments? The Chitta or mind-stuff, the Buddhi or determinative faculty, the Manas or mind, and the Indriyas or sense-organs.

These are the instruments for him to see the external world, and the identification of the Self with the instruments is what is called the ignorance of egoism. We say, "I am the mind," "I am thought," "I am angry," or "I am happy".

How can we be angry and how can we hate? We should identify ourselves with the Self that cannot change. If It is unchangeable, how can It be one moment happy, and one moment unhappy? It is formless, infinite, omnipresent.

What can change It? It is beyond all law. What can affect it? Nothing in the universe can produce an effect on It. Yet through ignorance, we identify ourselves with the mind-stuff, and think we feel pleasure or pain.

This Oneness of life, this Oneness of everything, is another great theme of the Vedanta,

We shall see how it demonstrates that all our misery comes through ignorance, and this ignorance is the idea of manifoldness, this separation between man and man, between nation and nation, between earth and moon, between moon and sun. Out of this idea of separation between atom and atom comes all misery.

But the Vedanta says this separation does not exist, it is not real. It is merely apparent, on the surface. In the heart of things there is Unity still. If you go below the surface, you find that Unity between man and man, between races and races, high and low, rich and poor, gods and men, and men and animals.

If you go deep enough, all will be seen as only variations of the One, and he who has attained to this conception of Oneness has no more delusion. What can delude him? He knows the reality of everything, the secret of everything. Where is there any more misery for him? What does he desire?

He has traced the reality of everything to the Lord, the Centre, the Unity of everything, and that is Eternal Existence, Eternal Knowledge, Eternal Bliss. Neither death nor disease, nor sorrow, nor misery, nor discontent is there.

All is Perfect Union and Perfect Bliss. For whom should he mourn then? In the Reality, there is no death, there is no misery; in the Reality, there is no one to mourn for, no one to be sorry for. He has penetrated everything, the Pure One, the Formless, the Bodiless, the Stainless.

He the Knower, He the Great Poet, the Self-Existent, He who is giving to everyone what he deserves. They grope in darkness who worship this ignorant world, the world that is produced out of ignorance, thinking of it as Existence, and those who live their whole lives in this world, and never find anything better or higher, are groping in still greater darkness.

But he who knows the secret of nature, seeing That which is beyond nature through the help of nature, he crosses death, and through the help of That which is beyond nature, he enjoys Eternal Bliss.

"Thou sun, who hast covered the Truth with thy golden disc, do thou remove the veil, so that I may see the Truth that is within thee. I have known the Truth that is within thee, I have known what is the real meaning of thy rays and thy glory and have seen That which shines in thee; the Truth in thee I see, and That which is within thee is within me, and I am That."

*

If then we are beyond all law, we must be omniscient, ever-blessed; all knowledge must be in us and all power and blessedness. Certainly. You are the omniscient. omnipresent being of the universe.

But of such beings can there be many? Can there be a hundred thousand millions of omnipresent beings? Certainly not. Then, what becomes of us all? You are only one; there is only one such Self, and that One Self is you.

Standing behind this little nature is what we call the Soul. There is only One Being, One Existence, the ever-blessed, the omnipresent, the omniscient, the birthless, deathless.

"Through His control the sky expands, through His control the air breathes, through His control the sun shines, and through His control all live. He is the Reality in nature, He is the Soul of your soul, nay, more, you are He, you are one with Him."

Wherever there are two, there is fear, there is danger, there is conflict, there is strife. When it is all One, who is there to hate, who is there to struggle with? When it is all He, with whom can you fight? T

his explains the true nature of life; this explains the true nature of being. this is perfection, and this is God. As long as you see the many, you are under delusion.

"In this world of many he who sees the One, in this everchanging world he who sees Him who never changes, as the Soul of his own soul, as his own Self, he is free, he is blessed, he has reached the goal."

Therefore know that thou art He; thou art the God of this universe, "Tat Tvam Asi" (That thou art).

All these various ideas that I am a man or a woman, or sick or healthy, or strong or weak, or that I hate or I love, or have a little power, are but hallucinations. Away with them!

What makes you weak? What makes you fear? You are the One Being in the universe. What frightens you? Stand up then and be free.

Know that every thought and word that weakens you in this world is the only evil that exists. Whatever makes men weak and fear is the only evil that should be shunned.

What can frighten you? If the suns come down, and the moons crumble into dust, and systems after systems are hurled into annihilation, what is that to you?

Stand as a rock; you are indestructible. You are the Self, the God of the universe. Say — "I am Existence Absolute, Bliss Absolute, Knowledge Absolute, I am He," and like a lion breaking its cage, break your chain and be free for ever.

What frightens you, what holds you down? Only ignorance and delusion; nothing else can bind you. You are the Pure One, the Ever-blessed.

Faith in God and in one's own Self is virtue; doubt is sin. Knowledge of oneness is virtue; seeing diversity is sin. The different scriptures only show the means of attaining virtue.

Two forces seem to be working throughout nature. One of these is constantly differentiating, and the other is as constantly unifying; the one making more and more for separate individuals, the other, as it were, bringing the individuals into a mass, bringing out sameness in the midst of all this differentiation. It seems that the action of these two forces enters into every department of nature and of human life.

On the physical plane, we always find the two forces most distinctly at work, separating the individuals, making them more and more distinct from other individuals, and again making them into species and classes, and bringing out similarities of expressions, and form. The same holds good as regards the social life of man.

Since the time when society began, these two forces have been at work, differentiating and unifying. Their action appears in various forms, and is called by various names, in different places, and at different times. But the essence is present in all, one making for differentiation, and the other for sameness; the one making for caste, and the other breaking it down; one making for classes and privileges, and the other destroying them.

The whole universe seems to be the battle-ground of these two forces. On the one hand, it is urged, that though this unifying process exists, we ought to resist it with all our might, because it leads towards death, that perfect unity is perfect annihilation, and that when the differentiating process that is at work in this universe ceases, the universe comes to an end. It is differentiation that causes the phenomena that are before us; unification would reduce them all to a homogeneous and lifeless matter.

Such a thing, of course, mankind wants to avoid. The same argument is applied to all the things and facts that we see around us. It is urged that even in physical body and social classification, absolute sameness would produce natural death and social death. Absolute sameness of thought and feeling would produce mental decay and degeneration.

Sameness, therefore, is to be avoided. This has been the argument on the one side, and it has been urged in every country and in various times, with only a change of language.

Practically it is the same argument which is urged by the Brahmins of India, when they want to uphold the divisions and castes, when they want to uphold the privileges of a certain portion of the community, against everybody else. The destruction of caste, they declare, would lead to destruction of society, and boldly they produce the historical fact that theirs has been the longest-lived society.

So they, with some show of force, appeal to this argument. With some show of authority they declare that that alone which makes the individual live the longest life must certainly be better than that which produces shorter lives.

On the other hand, the idea of oneness has had its advocates throughout all times. From the days of the Upanishads, the Buddhas, and Christs, and all other great preachers of religion, down to our present day, in the new political aspirations, and in the claims of the oppressed and the downtrodden, and of all those who find themselves bereft of privileges — comes out the one assertion of this unity and sameness.

The rational West is earnestly bent upon seeking out the rationality, the raison d' être of all its philosophy and its ethics. And you all know well that ethics cannot be derived from the mere sanction of any personage, however great and divine he may have been.

Such an explanation of the authority of ethics appeals no more to the highest of the world's thinkers. They want something more than human sanction for ethical and moral codes to be binding, they want some eternal principle of truth as the sanction of ethics.

And where is that eternal sanction to be found except in the only Infinite Reality that exists in you and in me and in all, in the Self, in the Soul? The infinite oneness of the Soul is the eternal sanction of all morality, that you and I are not only brothers — every literature voicing man's struggle towards freedom has preached that for you — but that you and I are really one.

This is the dictate of Indian philosophy. This oneness is the rationale of all ethics and all spirituality. Europe wants it today just as much as our downtrodden masses do, and this great principle is even now unconsciously forming the basis of all the latest political and social aspirations that are coming up in England, in Germany, in France, and in America.

And mark it, my friends, that in and through all the literature voicing man's struggle towards freedom, towards universal freedom, again and again you find the Indian Vedantic ideals coming out prominently. In some cases the writers do not know the source of their inspiration, in some cases they try to appear very original, and a few there are, bold and grateful enough to mention the source and acknowledge their indebtedness to it.

It is from the idea of the manifold that the ideas of virtue and vice have evolved. The more a man advances towards oneness, the more ideas of "I" and "you" subside, ideas from which all these pairs of opposites such as virtue and vice have originated.

When the idea that So-and-so is different from me comes to the mind, all other ideas of distinction begin to manifest, while with the complete realisation of oneness, no more grief or illusion remains for man, " — For him who sees oneness, where is there any grief or any delusion?"

Sin may be said to be the feeling of every kind of weakness. From this weakness spring jealousy, malice, and so forth.

Hence weakness is sin. The Self within is always shining forth resplendent. Turning away from that people say "I", "I", "I", with their attention held up by this material body, this queer cage of flesh and bones. This is the root of all weakness. From that habit only, the relative outlook on life has emerged in this world. The absolute Truth lies beyond that duality.

*

Mohammed found that Christianity was straying out from the Semitic fold and his teachings were to show what Christianity ought to be as a Semitic religion, that it should hold to one God. The Aryan idea that "I and my Father are one" disgusted and terrified him.

In reality the conception of the Trinity was a great advance over the dualistic idea of

Jehovah, who was for ever separate from man. The theory of incarnation is the first link in the chain of ideas leading to the recognition of the oneness of God and man.

God appearing first in one human form, then re-appearing at different times in other human forms, is at last recognised as being in every human form, or in all men. Monistic is the highest stage, monotheistic is a lower stage. Imagination will lead you to the highest even more rapidly and easily than reasoning.

In all religions we travel from a lesser to a higher truth, never from error to truth. There is a Oneness behind all creation, but minds are very various. 'That which exists is One, sages call It variously.'

What I mean is that one progresses from a smaller to a greater truth. The worst religions are only bad readings of the froth. One gets to understand bit by bit. Even devil-worship is but a perverted reading of the ever-true and immutable Brahman. Other phases have more or less of the truth in them. No form of religion possesses it entirely.

All that is meant by dying or being born is simply changes in the plane of vision. Neither do you move, nor does that move upon which you project your vision. You are the permanent, the unchangeable.

How can you come and go? It is impossible; you are omnipresent. The sky never moves, but the clouds move over the surface of the sky, and we may think that the sky itself moves, just as when you are in a railway train, you think the land is moving.

It is not so, but it is the train which is moving. You are where you are; these dreams, these various clouds move. One dream follows another without connection. There is no such thing as law or connection in this world, but we are thinking that there is a great deal of connection.

When this dream changes, another dream will seem quite as connected as this. When we dream, the things we see all seem to be connected; during the dream we never think they are incongruous; it is only when we wake that we see the want of connection.

When we wake from this dream of the world and compare it with the Reality, it will be found all incongruous nonsense, a mass of incongruity passing before us, we do not know whence or whither, but we know it will end; and this is called Maya, and is like masses of fleeting fleecy clouds.

They represent all this changing existence, and the sun itself, the unchanging, is you. When you look at that unchanging Existence from the outside, you call it God; and when you look at it from the inside, you call it yourself. It is but one.

There is no God separate from you, no God higher than you, the real "you". All the gods are little beings to you, all the ideas of God and Father in heaven are but your own reflection. God Himself is your image.

"God created man after His own image." That is wrong. Man creates God after his own image. That is right.

Throughout the universe we are creating gods after our own image. We create the god and fall down at his feet and worship him; and when this dream comes, we love it!

This is a good point to understand — that the sum and substance of this lecture is that there is but One Existence, and that One-Existence seen through different constitutions appears either as the earth, or heaven, or hell, or gods, or ghosts, or men, or demons, or world, or all these things.

But among these many, "He who sees that One in this ocean of death, he who sees that One Life in this floating universe, who realises that One who never changes, unto him belongs eternal peace; unto none else, unto none else."

"This earth is blissful ('sweet' is the literal translation) to all beings and all beings are sweet to this earth; they all help each other. And all the sweetness is the Atman, that effulgent, immortal One who is inside this earth."

Whose is this sweetness? How can there be any sweetness but He? That one sweetness is manifesting itself in various ways. Wherever there is any love, any sweetness in any human being, either in a saint or a sinner, either in an angel or a murderer, either in the body, mind, or the senses, it is He.

Physical enjoyments are but He, mental enjoyments are but He, spiritual enjoyments are but He. How can there be anything but He? How can there be twenty thousand gods and devils fighting with each other? Childish dreams!

Whatever is the lowest physical enjoyment is He, and the highest spiritual enjoyment is He. There is no sweetness but He. Thus says Yajnavalkya.

When you come to that state and look upon all things with the same eye, when you see even in the drunkard's pleasure in drink only that sweetness, then you have got the truth, and then alone you will know what happiness means, what peace means, what love means; and so long as toll make these vain distinctions, silly, childish, foolish superstitions, all sorts of misery will come.

But that immortal One, the effulgent One, He is inside the earth, it is all His sweetness, and the same sweetness is in the body.

This body is the earth, as it were, and inside all the powers of the body, all the enjoyments of the body, is He; the eyes see, the skin touches; what are all these enjoyments? That Self-effulgent One who is in the body, He is the Atman.

This world, so sweet to all beings, and every being so sweet to it, is but the Self-effulgent; the Immortal is the bliss in that world. In us also, He is that bliss. He is the Brahman.

"This air is so sweet to all beings, and all beings are so sweet to it. But He who is that Self-effulgent Immortal Being in the air — is also in this body. He is expressing Himself as the life of all beings. This sun is so sweet to all beings. All beings are so sweet to this sun. He who is the Self-effulgent Being in the sun, we reflect Him as the smaller light. What can be there but His reflection? He is in the body, and it is His reflection which makes us see the light. This moon is so sweet to all, and every one is so sweet to the moon, but that Self-effulgent and Immortal One who is the soul of that moon, He is in us expressing Himself as mind. This lightning is so beautiful, every one is so sweet to the lightning, but the Self-effulgent and Immortal One is the soul of this lightning, and is also in us, because all is that Brahman. The Atman, the Self, is the king of all beings."

These ideas are very helpful to men; they are for meditation. For instance, meditate on the earth; think of the earth and at the same time know that we have That which is in the earth, that both are the same. Identify the body with the earth, and identify the soul with the Soul behind. Identify the air with the soul that is in the air and that is in me. They are all one, manifested in different forms. To realise this unity is the end and aim of all meditation.

One principle the Vedanta philosophy lays down — and that, the Vedanta claims, is to be found in every religion in the world — is that man is divine, that all this which we see around us is the outcome of that consciousness of the divine.

Everything that is strong, and good, and powerful in human nature is the outcome of that divinity, and though potential in many, there is no difference between man and man essentially, all being alike divine. There is, as it were, an infinite ocean behind, and you and I are so many waves, coming out of that infinite ocean; and each one of us is trying his best to manifest that infinite outside.

So, potentially, each one of us has that infinite ocean of Existence, Knowledge, and Bliss as our birthright, our real nature; and the difference between us is caused by the greater or lesser power to manifest that divine.

Therefore the Vedanta lays down that each man should be treated not as what he manifests, but as what he stands for. Each human being stands for the divine, and, therefore, every teacher should be helpful, not by condemning man, but by helping him to call forth the divinity that is within him.

It also teaches that all the vast mass of energy that we see displayed in society and in every plane of action is really from inside out; and, therefore, what is called inspiration by other sects, the Vedantist begs the liberty to call the expiration of man.

Consciously or unconsciously, every man is trying to unfold that divinity. At the same time it does not quarrel with other sects; the Vedanta has no quarrel with those who do not understand this divinity of man.

Now, this idea, claims the Vedanta, is to be found in all religions, whether in India or outside of it; only, in some of them, the idea is expressed through mythology, and in others, through symbology. The Vedanta claims that there has not been one religious inspiration, one manifestation of the divine man, however great, but it has been the expression of that infinite oneness in human nature; and all that we call ethics and morality and doing good to others is also but the manifestation of this oneness.

There are moments when every man feels that he is one with the universe, and he rushes forth to express it, whether he knows it or not. This expression of oneness is what we call love and sympathy, and it is the basis of all our ethics and morality. This is summed up in the Vedanta philosophy by the celebrated aphorism, Tat Tvam Asi, "Thou art That".

To every man, this is taught: Thou art one with this Universal Being, and, as such, every soul that exists is your soul; and everybody that exists is your body; and in hurting anyone, you hurt yourself, in loving anyone, you love yourself.

As soon as a current of hatred is thrown outside, whomsoever else it hurts, it also hurts yourself; and if love comes out from you, it is bound to come back to you. For I am the universe; this universe is my body. I am the Infinite, only I am not conscious of it now; but I am struggling to get this consciousness of the Infinite, and perfection will be reached when full consciousness of this Infinite comes.